Devotio1

BIBLE-BASED
Devotional for New Moms

You Can Overcome Postpartum Emotions and Newborn Stress with Guided, Weekly Devotions That Bring Peace in
Just Minutes a Day

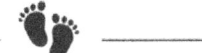

PUBLISHED BY: Julie Whitecotton

© Copyright Julie Whitecotton 2025
- All rights reserved.

Julie Whitecotton

The content contained within this book may not be reproduced, duplicated or transmitted without direct written permission from the author or the publisher.

Under no circumstances will any blame or legal responsibility be held against the publisher, or author, for any damages, reparation, or monetary loss due to the information contained within this book. Either directly or indirectly. You are responsible for your own choices, actions, and results.

Legal Notice:

This book is copyright protected. This book is only for personal use. You cannot amend, distribute, sell, use, quote or paraphrase any part, or the content within this book, without the consent of the author or publisher.

Disclaimer Notice:

Please note the information contained within this document is for educational and entertainment purposes only. All effort has been executed to present accurate, up to date, and reliable, complete information. No warranties of any kind are declared or implied. Readers acknowledge that the author is not engaging in the rendering of legal, financial, medical or professional advice. The content within this book has been derived from various sources. Please consult a licensed professional before attempting any techniques outlined in this book.

By reading this document, the reader agrees that under no circumstances is the author responsible for any losses, direct or indirect, which are incurred as a result of the use of the information contained within this document, including, but not limited to, errors, omissions, or inaccuracies.

Note to the Reader

This devotional is intended for spiritual encouragement and personal reflection. It is not a substitute for medical advice, diagnosis, mental-health support, or professional counseling. Every mother's health and journey is unique—please consult a qualified healthcare provider, physician, or licensed professional regarding any questions or concerns related to pregnancy, postpartum recovery, or your child's health and development.

Scripture references are provided for personal study and inspiration. While this book offers faith-based guidance, it does not guarantee specific outcomes in emotional, physical, or spiritual well-being. The author encourages all readers to make prayerful decisions, seek wisdom from trusted professionals, and care for themselves with patience, grace, and compassion.

Julie Whitecotton

Color-Me Prayer Cards for New Moms

As a special gift, you get access to **beautiful, printable Prayer Cards** designed just for new moms. Each card features:

- A **Bible verse** chosen for comfort, strength, and encouragement
- A **simple, soothing coloring background** (florals, patterns, soft lines)
- Designs that are perfect for your journal, fridge, mirror, diaper bag, or nursery

These cards are created to help you **pause**, breathe, pray, and reconnect with God—
even on days when quiet time feels impossible.

You can color them for personal reflection, use them as bookmarks, tape them to your mirror, or share them with a friend who needs encouragement.

☞ **Download your free set at:**

https://morningvalleypress.com/Prayer-Cards

Introduction

Becoming a mother truly changes everything: your schedule, your priorities, even the way your heart beats. The moment you hold your baby for the first time, it's like the world shifts. There's a love you've never felt before, mixed with wonder, responsibility, and the quiet question every new mom asks: "Am I really ready for this?" And that's okay. God meets you right there in the excitement, the exhaustion, the joy, and the unspoken worries.

This devotional is for you, the mom who wants God to be part of every step of this new journey. Over the next 52 weeks, you'll find gentle encouragement from Scripture, reminders of God's steady presence, and simple, practical ways to strengthen both your faith and your heart. Whether you're awake at 2 a.m. rocking your baby, drinking coffee before the house wakes up, or catching a breath during nap time, these pages are meant to meet you right where you are.

You don't have to be a perfect mom to be the mom God chose. He's not looking for flawless performance. He's looking for your heart. When you're tired, He offers rest. When you're unsure, He gives wisdom. When you feel unnoticed, He reminds you that He's been walking with you since the very beginning.

Think of this year as a journey, one where motherhood and faith grow together. Let God's peace steady you, let His love surround you, and let His grace carry you through every win and every hard moment. You are not alone. The same God who placed this child in your arms will give you everything you need to care for them.

So, take a slow breath, settle your heart, and step into this year with hope. These next 52 weeks are an invitation to a rhythm of grace, growth, and renewal as you walk closely with the One who entrusted you with this precious little life.

Table of Contents:

Note to the Reader 3

Color-Me Prayer Cards for New Moms 4

A New Beginning 1
Rest for the Weary 4
Finding Joy in the Chaos 7
Grace Upon Grace 10
The Strength Within 13
Nourishing Your Soul 17
The Gift of Small Moments 20
When You Feel Alone 23
Trusting God with Your Child 26
The Power of Prayer 29
Peace in the Unknown 32
Learning to Let Go 35
Celebrating Progress, ... 38
Not Perfection 38
Trusting God's Timing 41
Grace for Today 44
Peace in the Chaos 47
Anchored in Hope 50
Strong Foundations 53
Wisdom in Waiting 56
Walking by Faith 59
Compassion in Motion 62
The Beauty of Patience 65
Joy in Service 68
Faith Over Fear 71
Love That Never Fails 74
Strength in Surrender 77
Finding Beauty in the Ordinary 80
God's Faithfulness Never Fails 83
The Gift of Gentleness 86
When You Feel Overwhelmed 89
God's Perfect Provision 92
Holding Onto Peace 95
Finding Balance in a 98
Busy Season 98
The Blessing of Community 101
Blessed Beyond Measure 104
Rest in His Grace 107

Harvest of Blessings 110
Give Thanks Always 113
Joy in Every Season 116
Be a Light 119
Faithful and True 122
God's Love Endures 125
Hope Shines Bright 128
Guided by His Light 131
Moments of Renewal 134
Steadfast in Spirit 137
Overflowing with Gratitude 140
Grace-Filled Growth 143
The Power of Perseverance 146
Strength in Unity 149
A Heart of Joy 152
A Year of Grace 155
    Closing 158

A New Beginning

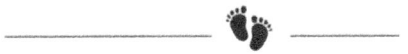

"See, I am doing a new thing! Now it springs up; do you not perceive it?"
-Isaiah 43:19

When your baby arrived, something inside you shifted forever. It's amazing how one tiny person can change your whole world in an instant. All the waiting, the nerves, the long nights, the wondering how life would feel, it all became real the moment you held that little one in your arms. And honestly, it's okay if you've already discovered that motherhood is a swirl of emotions. One moment you're smiling, the next you're crying, and sometimes you're not even sure why. That's part of the beauty and vulnerability of this season.

God is doing something new in you, too. Motherhood isn't just about learning to care for a baby; it's also about how God gently shapes *you* through every feeding, every diaper change, and every sleepy prayer whispered in the dark. He uses these small, everyday moments to stretch your patience, soften your heart, and strengthen your faith. You may feel overwhelmed at times, but you're not walking this path alone.

Julie Whitecotton

Remember this: you are caring for your baby, but your Heavenly Father is caring for *you*. When your thoughts start spiraling, call on Him. When you're exhausted beyond words, let His presence hold you. He isn't just giving you a new season. He's giving you new strength, new grace, and new hope for tomorrow. Nothing about this journey surprises Him. He chose you to be this child's mother, and He promises to walk with you through every moment, big or small.

Prayer:

Lord, thank You for the gift of this new beginning. Help me step into motherhood with faith, even when I feel unsure. On the days when I question myself, remind me that You have already equipped me for this calling. Fill my home and my heart with Your peace and teach me to lean on You through every joy and every tear. Amen.

Challenge of the Week:

Pay attention to one moment this week where you can clearly sense God's presence, maybe it's a peaceful pause, a kind word, or strength you didn't know you had. Write it down as a reminder that you're not walking this alone.

Mom Tip of the Week:

Please don't try to carry everything by yourself. Let someone bring you a meal, fold the laundry, or run an errand. This is a season of healing and bonding, and rest is part of your calling, not something to feel guilty about.

Julie Whitecotton

Rest for the Weary

"Come to me, all you who are weary and burdened, and I will give you rest."
-Matthew 11:28

If there's one thing motherhood teaches quickly, it's how deeply tired a person can feel. There are nights when you're awake more than you sleep, and days when you look at the clock wondering how it's somehow still morning. Your body feels worn, your mind is stretched, and your heart carries more responsibility than you ever imagined. Sometimes you wish you could pause life long enough to catch your breath.

But Jesus didn't wait for you to be well-rested before He made His invitation. He said, *"Come to Me."* Not *when you finally sleep*, not *when things settle down*, not *when you have it all together.* Come as you are, tired, overwhelmed, messy bun and all.

He wasn't only talking to the physically tired. He was speaking to anyone whose soul feels heavy... and that includes moms who feel stretched thin by constant needs and never-ending to-dos. The beautiful thing is that His rest isn't limited to quiet mornings or long naps. His rest can find you right there in the rocking chair at 2 a.m., over the sink full of bottles, or on the couch with a baby sleeping on your chest. It comes in a deep breath, a whispered prayer, or a moment where you let yourself be held by Him.

Remember, even Jesus stepped away from the noise to rest and pray. If the Son of God needed moments to recharge, then it's okay for you to need them, too. Strength doesn't come from powering through. It comes from leaning into the One who understands every tear, every ache, and every weary sigh.

You don't have to carry everything today. Let God meet you right where you are. Let Him refill what has been emptied. The same Jesus who calms storms with a word can calm the storm inside your tired heart, too.

Julie Whitecotton

Prayer:

Jesus, you see how tired I am, not just in my body, but deep in my soul. Thank You for inviting me to come to You just as I am. Teach me how to rest in You, even in the middle of busy days and long nights. Help me release the pressure I put on myself and breathe in Your peace. Restore me from the inside out. Amen.

Challenge of the Week:

Find five quiet minutes each day, even if it's while feeding your baby or sitting in the bathroom, and breathe. Close your eyes and whisper, *"Lord, I rest in You."* Let that moment reset your heart.

Mom Tip of the Week:

When your baby sleeps, try to rest too, even if it's just lying down for a few minutes. The world won't fall apart, but your spirit will feel the difference. A rested mom can love more freely than an exhausted one.

Finding Joy in the Chaos

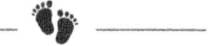

"The joy of the Lord is your strength."
- Nehemiah 8:10

The early weeks of motherhood can feel like a whirlwind, with feeding around the clock, endless laundry, and moments when you look in the mirror and barely recognize the tired face staring back. It's easy to wonder where joy fits into all of this. Sometimes it feels like joy belongs to a calmer season... a quieter season... a season where you actually sleep.

But God's joy doesn't wait for things to be neat or peaceful. His joy meets you right where you are, right in the middle of the noise, the mess, and the moments you're just trying to hold it all together. Think about those little flashes of beauty that sneak into your day: the way your baby's tiny fingers curl around yours, the unexpected giggle that melts your exhaustion, the warm weight of a sleeping child against your heart. Those moments might feel small, but they're sacred reminders that joy is still here.

Julie Whitecotton

Joy isn't pretending everything is perfect. It's choosing to see God's goodness even when your day feels completely undone. It's the quiet decision to look for Him in the ordinary places, in the deep breath you didn't know you needed, in the smile that surprises you, in the moment you feel just a little stronger than you did yesterday.

Every time you pause to thank God for one small blessing, you give His joy permission to slip into the cracks of your day and lift you. And that joy? That's where your strength comes from. Not from having everything together, but from knowing God is with you, even in the chaos.

So today, let yourself notice the sweetness tucked inside the mess. Laugh when your baby makes a silly sound. Smile at the tiny victories. Let the joy of the Lord be the steady strength that carries you through the moments that feel heavy and the ones that feel holy.

Prayer:

Lord, thank You for the kind of joy that doesn't depend on everything being calm or perfect. Help me notice Your goodness in the middle of my messy, beautiful days. When I start to feel overwhelmed, remind me that Your joy is what strengthens me and holds me steady. Fill my heart today with a joy that only You can give. Amen.

Challenge of the Week:

Each night before bed, write down three things that made you smile, even if they lasted only a second. Let gratitude become a gentle way to close your day.

Mom Tip of the Week:

Snap a picture of something real, not staged, your baby laughing beside a pile of laundry, or the messy kitchen after a day of trying your best. One day, you'll look back and see how beautiful this season truly was.

Julie Whitecotton

Grace Upon Grace

*"From His fullness we have all received,
grace upon grace."*
- John 1:16

If there's one thing almost every mom wrestles with, it's the pressure to get everything right. You want to respond with patience, keep your home in order, and somehow meet every need before anyone even asks. But real life doesn't always go that smoothly. There are days when you lose your temper, cry in the bathroom, or feel like you're failing at things you thought would come naturally.

But this is exactly where God's Word whispers hope: His grace doesn't wait until you've earned it. His grace pours in right when you feel empty, weak, or overwhelmed. It covers the moments you wish you could redo, the words you didn't mean to say, and the days you feel like you're falling apart. His grace isn't fragile; it's abundant, overflowing, and tailor-made for seasons just like this.

Motherhood isn't a performance; it's a journey of growth. Just as your baby is learning something new every day, so are you. You're learning to trust God more deeply... to release the need for control... to forgive yourself... and to rest in mercy instead of perfection.

Comparison and guilt may try to creep in, but God's grace is larger than your mistakes and stronger than your doubts.

Permit yourself to be human. You don't have to pretend or push yourself to impossible standards. The same God who formed your baby with such care is also forming new strength, patience, and peace within you. His grace meets you in the rocking chair at 3 a.m., in the tears you wipe from your eyes, and even in the messiest moments of your day.

You are held. You are covered. Not just once but again and again. Grace upon grace.

Prayer:

Father, thank You for the endless grace You pour over me. On the days I feel stretched thin or not enough, remind me that *You* are enough for both me and my child. Teach me to give grace freely to myself, to my baby, and to those around me. Let Your mercy wash over my heart and refresh me with new strength each morning. Amen.

Challenge of the Week:
When guilt or frustration starts to rise, pause and speak this truth out loud: "God's grace is enough for me." Let those words gently shift your heart from pressure to peace.

Mom Tip of the Week:
If your day starts to feel heavy, step outside for a moment, even if it's just to the porch or the doorway. Feel the fresh air, breathe slowly, and let the quiet remind you that grace grows in the pauses, not in the rush.

The Strength Within

"I can do all things through Christ who strengthens me."
- Philippians 4:13

Motherhood has a way of exposing both your limits and your hidden strength. There are moments when you feel like you're running on empty, you're tired, unsure, stretched thin, and wondering how you're supposed to keep going. Yet somehow... You do. Somehow, there's just enough strength for the next diaper, the next feeding, the next long night. And that "somehow" isn't luck, it's Christ in you.

The same God who shaped the stars and breathed life into creation is the One holding you steady in the quiet, unseen moments: when you're rocking a fussy baby at 3 a.m., when tears sting your eyes for reasons you can't even name, when your patience feels worn down to nothing. His strength doesn't always feel like a burst of energy. Often it looks like the simple ability to take one more step, whisper one more prayer, show love one more time, even when you feel completely poured out.

Julie Whitecotton

God isn't asking you to be superhuman. He's inviting you to lean on Him to stop pushing through in your own power and instead let His strength fill the spaces where you feel weak. When you pause, breathe, and turn your heart toward Him, He meets you right there.

He gives you strength that carries you through the day... not all at once, but moment by moment.

You were never meant to do motherhood alone. God chose *you* for this baby on purpose, not because you're perfect, but because His strength shines beautifully in your weakness. Every day you show up with love, even when it's hard, you're living out the truth of this verse. You are not failing. You are being held.

Prayer:

Lord, thank You for being my strength when I feel weak and overwhelmed. When my energy runs low or my confidence fades, remind me to lean into You instead of trying to manage everything on my own. Fill me with Your peace and power today. Help me face whatever comes with the assurance that You are with me in every moment. Amen.

Challenge of the Week:

Each morning, before you start your day, speak this simple truth aloud: "I am strong in the Lord." Let those words settle in your heart and remind you where your strength truly comes from.

Mom Tip of the Week:

When you feel your energy dipping, take a moment to hydrate, stretch, or breathe deeply. Sometimes a small physical reset opens your heart to receive the spiritual strength God is offering.

Julie Whitecotton

A Small Way to Pay the Blessing Forward

Thank you so much for purchasing and reading this devotional. You could have chosen from dozens of other books, yet you picked this one—and I am deeply grateful you joined me on this journey.

If this book has encouraged you, I'd love to ask one small favor: would you take a moment to leave a review on the platform where you purchased it? Your words are more than just feedback—they become a guiding light for other mothers searching for hope, peace, and encouragement in this season.

When you share your experience, you're not only supporting me as an independent author, but you're also blessing another mom who might be walking through the same joys and challenges you've faced. Think of your review as a way to pass along encouragement, like holding out a hand to someone coming up the path behind you.

Thank you again for choosing this book. May your journey of motherhood continue to be filled with God's presence, peace, and joy.

>> Leave a review on Amazon US <<

>> Leave a review on Amazon UK <<

If you are reading this in a paperback/hardcover copy, please go to your Amazon page. Click orders. Find this purchase and leave a review.

Nourishing Your Soul

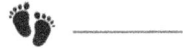

"Man shall not live by bread alone, but by every word that comes from the mouth of God."
-Matthew 4:4

As a new mom, so much of your day revolves around nourishing your baby. You track feedings, wash bottles, measure ounces, and celebrate every sign of growth. You're constantly pouring yourself out, making sure your little one has everything they need to thrive. But in all that giving, it's surprisingly easy to forget that *your soul* needs nourishment too.

There's a quiet hunger inside you not for food, but for peace... for strength... for a sense of grounding when the days blur together. And the truth is, only God can feed that part of you. A few honest moments with Him, even the smallest ones, can fill your spirit in ways sleep and coffee never could.

God's Word is more than information; it's nourishment for a weary heart. It reminds you who you are when you feel like you're losing pieces of yourself in the busyness of newborn life. It steadies your mind when emotions are all over the place. It brings back perspective when you feel overwhelmed.

And here's the comforting part: God isn't waiting for you to carve out a perfect, silent hour. He knows your season. He sees the diaper changes, the dishes, the interrupted naps. He's ready to meet you in tiny moments, a verse read while the baby naps, a whispered prayer while folding onesies, worship music humming in the background of a noisy home. He loves showing up in the ordinary.

Your soul matters as much as your baby's well-being. When you stay connected to God's Word, your heart becomes a place of peace that spills over into your home. His truth becomes the anchor that steadies you when doubt or exhaustion tries to pull you under. And the more you let Him speak into your life, the more you'll notice His strength and joy flowing out through you right into your little one's world.

Prayer:

Lord, thank You for Your Word that nourishes me in ways nothing else can. Help me remember to meet You in the small moments of my day, even when life feels chaotic. Remind me that my spiritual health matters, and fill my heart with Your peace and presence. Let Your truth sustain me and help me grow as I care for my precious child. Amen.

Challenge of the Week:

Choose one simple verse each morning and sit with it for a moment. Write it on a sticky note, place it by your bed, or save it on your phone. When you start feeling drained or scattered, pause and read it again.

Mom Tip of the Week:

Keep a Bible or devotional near the place you nurse or rock your baby. Even a few quiet verses during those moments can turn a tired day into a peaceful one.

Julie Whitecotton

The Gift of Small Moments

"Be still, and know that I am God."
-Psalm 46:10

It's natural to think the biggest parts of motherhood are the big "firsts": the first smile, the first giggle, the first wobbling steps. Those moments are precious, of course, and they'll stay with you forever. But what many moms discover, often without realizing it at first, is that the real beauty of this season is tucked quietly into the small moments, the ones no one else sees but you.

It's found in the peaceful weight of your baby sleeping against your chest. In the early-morning hush when the world hasn't quite woken up and you're rocking your little one in the soft light of dawn. In the way your baby's tiny fingers curl around yours. In the whispered prayers you breathe over your child when the house is still. These moments are so quick, but they carry a kind of sacred tenderness that stays with you long after the day is over.

Our culture pushes us to move faster, do more, and achieve constantly. But God often speaks in the quiet... in the stillness... in those calm in-between moments when your heart finally slows down enough to hear Him. You don't need a mountaintop experience or a perfectly quiet morning to feel close to Him. He meets you right in the middle of the toys on the floor, the unwashed dishes, and the soft lull of your baby's breathing.

This season is holy ground, not because everything is perfect, but because God is present in every detail. Try not to rush through it, even when it feels overwhelming. One day, you'll look back and realize how meaningful these little pieces of your day truly were.

When you slow down just long enough to notice God's hand in the ordinary, you begin to find a peace that no routine or schedule could ever give.

Prayer:

Father, help me slow down and notice You in the middle of my day. Open my eyes to the quiet, simple moments that show Your love and goodness. Teach me not to rush through this precious season, but to treasure the beauty right in front of me. Let my heart rest in Your presence and find peace in the small things. Amen.

Challenge of the Week:

Once each day, pause and thank God for one small moment, something gentle and ordinary that you might have missed if you hadn't slowed down.

Mom Tip of the Week:

Start a little "tiny blessings" journal. Each day, write down one simple joy: a sweet look, a funny sound, a peaceful moment. These small memories will one day be your most treasured keepsakes.

When You Feel Alone

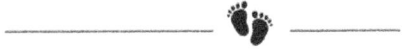

"The Lord your God goes with you; He will never leave you nor forsake you."
-Deuteronomy 31:6

Motherhood is full of beautiful moments, the sweet smiles, the soft snuggles, the tiny hands reaching out for you. Yet even with all the love, it can still feel surprisingly lonely. There are long nights when everyone else in the house is asleep except you and the baby. There are days when the routine feels repetitive, and you start to wonder if anyone really sees the weight you're carrying.

People can surround you and still feel unseen. That kind of loneliness hits deep.

But here's the gentle truth you need to hold close: *God sees you*. Not just the polished parts, He sees the messy bun, the tired eyes, the quiet tears, the moments when you're trying your best and still feel like you're falling short. And he's not distant. He's right there in the stillness with you.

When you're sitting in the dim light, rocking your baby back to sleep, and your thoughts begin to wander, He is there steady, present, whispering peace into places you didn't even know were aching. God doesn't wait for you to feel strong or joyful before He draws near. He steps into your weariness with compassion, understanding the tired that goes beyond the body and settles into the soul.

Even the most loving, devoted mother needs connection. Ask God to guide you toward people who will truly understand your season, maybe another new mom, a trusted friend, or a small church group. You weren't created to walk this journey alone.

But even on the days when human connection feels far away, you are *never* abandoned. The God who holds the stars in place is holding you, too. His presence is your safest place, your steady companion, and your unfailing comfort. You don't have to carry motherhood alone. He is with you every hour, every tear, every quiet moment.

Prayer:

Lord, when loneliness settles into my heart, remind me that You are right here with me. Help me feel Your presence in the quiet moments and the long nights. Fill the empty spaces in my heart with Your comfort and peace. Thank You for never leaving me, even when I struggle to sense You. Hold me close today. Amen.

Challenge of the Week:

Reach out to just one mom with a text, a message, or a simple "thinking of you." Sometimes the smallest connection can remind both of you that you're not walking this journey alone.

Mom Tip of the Week:

Consider joining a small group at church or a local moms' circle. Being around others who understand your season can slowly turn isolation into connection and loneliness into genuine friendship.

Julie Whitecotton

Trusting God with Your Child

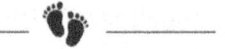

"For this child I prayed, and the Lord has granted me what I asked of Him."

-1 Samuel 1:27

From the moment you found out you were expecting, something in your heart shifted. You began praying, maybe quietly at first, maybe with tears for this little life growing inside you. You prayed for health, protection, and a future filled with purpose. And those prayers didn't stop once your baby arrived. If anything, they've grown deeper and more urgent.

It's only natural for a mother to feel fiercely protective. You want to guard your child from every hurt, every sickness, every uncertainty. But in those quiet moments when worry creeps in, God gently reminds you of something both comforting and profound: He loves your baby even more than you do. As unbelievable as that sounds, it's true. Your child belonged to Him before they were ever placed in your arms.

Hannah's story in Scripture is such a beautiful picture of this kind of trust. She prayed and longed for a child, and when God answered her prayer, she dedicated little Samuel back to the Lord. Not because she loved him less, but because she understood that children are gifts entrusted to us, held ultimately by God Himself.

Trusting God with your child doesn't mean you stop caring or stop being protective. It means you stop carrying fear alone. When worries wake you up at night, remember: God doesn't sleep. His watchful care never ends. You can rest because He is always awake.

There will be days when things don't go according to your plans, fevers, delays, and unexpected challenges. In those moments, instead of gripping your fear tighter, try opening your hands in prayer. Whisper your anxieties to the One who already stands in your child's future. He sees what you can't. He guides where you cannot go. And He loves with a depth we'll never fully understand.

Your role is important, but you were never meant to carry the full weight of motherhood alone. Trust Him. He is faithful, and He is already caring for your child in ways you cannot see.

Prayer:

Lord, thank You for this precious life You've entrusted to me. When worry rises in my heart, remind me that You are the ultimate protector and provider. Teach me to surrender my fears and trust Your loving care over my child's life. Strengthen my faith, and help me rest in the truth that You have beautiful plans for my baby. Amen.

Challenge of the Week:

Each day this week, pray specifically over your baby, speak blessings over their health, their future, and their heart. Trust that God hears every single word.

Mom Tip of the Week:

When anxiety begins to rise, pause and speak Scripture out loud over your child. Let God's Word, spoken through your voice, fill your home with peace and reassurance.

The Power of Prayer

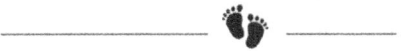

"Pray without ceasing."
                                        -1 Thessalonians 5:17

Motherhood will give you more reasons to pray than anything else ever has. You'll pray for strength when the night feels long... for patience when you're stretched thin... for peace when anxiety creeps in... and for rest when you can barely keep your eyes open. Some days, your prayers will spill out in full sentences. Other days, they'll look like a deep sigh, a tear slipping down your face, or a quiet "Lord, please help me." And the beautiful truth is *God hears them all.*

Prayer isn't about sounding polished. It's about staying connected. It's breathing in His presence when you feel empty and letting Him hold you in moments when you don't have the words. God invites you to bring everything to Him: the frustration, the wonder, the fear, the gratitude, and even the moments when your heart feels too tired to speak.

Your days may not leave much room for long, uninterrupted prayer times, and that's okay. You can pray while you change diapers, fold onesies, drive to appointments, or rock your baby to sleep. You can pray in fragments half half-sentences, whispered thoughts, and they still reach the throne of God.

As you begin to turn your everyday thoughts into quiet conversations with Him, something shifts. His peace settles deeper. His presence feels closer. Prayer stops feeling like another task and becomes the gentle rhythm of your day, the steady backdrop that keeps your heart anchored when life feels overwhelming.

Every prayer, no matter how small, invites God into your story. When you pray, you're not just asking for help, you're staying close to the One who loves you deeply. You're saying, *"Lord, I can't do this without You."* And He responds, *"You don't have to. I'm right here."*

Prayer:

Heavenly Father, thank You for listening to me, even when my prayers are messy or quiet. Teach me to turn to You first in joy, in exhaustion, and in worry. Help me stay connected to Your heart throughout my day, and let Your peace fill every room of my home. Amen.

Challenge of the Week:

Each time worry tries to settle in your mind, stop and pray one simple sentence: "God, I trust You." Let that small act turn your anxieties into moments of surrender.

Mom Tip of the Week:

As you rock or feed your baby, speak blessings over them. These gentle, consistent prayers become seeds of faith planted quietly now, growing beautifully over time.

Julie Whitecotton

Peace in the Unknown

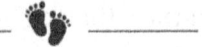

"You will keep in perfect peace those whose minds are steadfast, because they trust in You."
-Isaiah 26:3

Motherhood is full of constant change. One week your baby sleeps well, and the next week everything is upside down again. Routines shift, milestones come unexpectedly, and new challenges seem to show up just when you think you've finally found your rhythm. It's easy to start asking yourself, *what's coming next? Will tonight be another long night? Am I doing this right? What if I can't handle what's ahead?*

Those thoughts can stir up so much worry. But God reminds us that peace doesn't come from having all the answers; it comes from trusting the One who already does.

God's peace isn't delicate or easily shaken. It's strong and steady, like an anchor in stormy water. When your mind starts spinning with "what ifs," He invites you to turn your thoughts back toward Him. You don't need to understand every detail of what tomorrow holds. You need to rest in the truth that God is already there preparing, guiding, and working things together for your good.

The same God who carried you through yesterday will carry you through today... and tomorrow... and every day after.

As you fix your heart on Christ, peace begins to show up in surprising places in the middle of a sleepless night, while holding your baby through a difficult moment, during appointments that tug at your heart, or in seasons of waiting where you long for answers. God's peace doesn't remove all uncertainty, but it quiets your soul even while the world around you feels unpredictable.

You can breathe deeply knowing this: even in the unknown, you are held by a God who never loses control. His peace is not the absence of hard things; it's the presence of His unshakable love right in the middle of them.

Prayer:

Lord, thank You for being my peace in every season, especially when life feels uncertain. When worry starts to rise in my heart, quiet my thoughts and remind me that You are in control. Help me keep my mind centered on You and trust that You are guiding every step I take. Fill my home with Your calm and my heart with Your steady love. Amen.

Challenge of the Week:

Whenever you start to feel anxious about something out of your control, pause, take a slow breath, and whisper: **"I trust You, Lord."** Repeat it until your heart feels lighter.

Mom Tip of the Week:

Create a simple bedtime ritual just for you, a short prayer, a deep breathing moment, or a verse to reflect on. Ending your day with peace helps you wake with fresh strength and a quieter heart.

Learning to Let Go

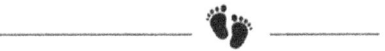

"Cast all your anxiety on Him because He cares for you."

- 1 Peter 5:7

One of the first lessons motherhood teaches is this: there is so much you *can't* control. You can't control when your baby will sleep, how your body heals, or how smoothly the day will go, no matter how carefully you plan it. You try your best and still, things shift, unravel, or take unexpected turns. And when they do, it's easy to feel frustration rising, guilt creeping in, or anxiety settling heavily on your heart.

But tucked inside those overwhelming moments is a gentle invitation from God: *Let go.*

Letting go doesn't mean you stop caring or become less intentional. It means you stop trying to carry burdens that were never meant to rest on your shoulders. And as a mom, that can feel hard because loving a child so deeply makes you want to control everything that touches their life.

Julie Whitecotton

When Peter wrote "cast your cares," the word he used meant to *throw* to release something completely, not pass it off timidly. God isn't asking you to manage your worries; He's inviting you to drop them into His hands. Fully. Completely. Without taking them back five minutes later.

Why? Because He cares for you deeply, personally, tenderly. He cares about your child. He cares about your healing. He cares about the details of your day. And His shoulders are strong enough to carry what yours were never meant to hold.

Letting go is rarely a one-time thing. It's a daily choice, sometimes a moment-by-moment one. You may find yourself releasing fear about your baby's health today, and then again tomorrow... and again next week. That's okay. Each time you choose to surrender instead of cling, your faith grows a little stronger. Little by little, you'll feel your heart lighten as you trust Him more fully.

The same God who carried you through pregnancy, labor, birth, and every moment since He's still carrying you. You don't have to be in control. You have to be in His care. And that is the safest, most peaceful place you could ever be.

Prayer:

Lord, help me let go of the things I cannot control. You know the worries I carry and how tightly I hold onto them. Take my fear, my stress, and my desire to have everything figured out. Fill those spaces with Your peace. Remind me each day that You care for me and my child more deeply than I can understand. Amen.

Challenge of the Week:

Write down three worries you've been holding onto. Pray over each one, then fold or tear the paper as a simple, physical reminder that you are releasing them into God's hands.

Mom Tip of the Week:

Simplify where you can routines, chores, and expectations. A peaceful mom helps create a peaceful home, and calm often starts by removing the unnecessary things that crowd your space and your mind.

Julie Whitecotton

Celebrating Progress, Not Perfection

*"Let us not become weary in doing good,
for at the proper time we will reap
a harvest if we do not give up."*
- Galatians 6:9

It's so easy, especially as a new mom, to measure your worth by what you accomplish in a day. You might catch yourself thinking, *Did I get the house clean? Did the baby sleep well? Did I keep everything together today?* But God isn't asking you to perform or keep up a perfect routine. He's inviting you to keep going one loving, faithful step at a time.

Every diaper you change, every midnight feeding, every moment you hold your baby close, it's all part of the good work God has placed in your hands. These small acts might not look impressive on the outside, but in God's eyes, they are seeds of love and faithfulness that will one day bloom into something beautiful. You are sowing into your child's life in ways you may not fully see yet.

And while your baby is growing, you are growing too. Motherhood is shaping you into a woman with deeper strength, softer compassion, and stronger faith. Some days, your progress might feel invisible, like nothing is changing, like you're stuck on repeat, but God often works beneath the surface long before we see the fruit. The goal was never perfection. The goal is transformation. And transformation takes time.

When discouragement creeps in, pause and look back. Think about the things that once overwhelmed you that now come naturally. Think about the prayers God has answered and the grace He's given you along the way. Celebrate those moments, even the smallest steps forward. God sees every effort, every sacrifice, every tear. And He is pleased with your faithfulness.

Perfection isn't what He asks of you. Persistence is. Showing up with love is. Trusting Him with your growth is. That's where the real beauty of motherhood lives in progress that is slow, steady, and covered in grace.

Prayer:

Lord, thank You for reminding me that progress is enough. Help me notice the ways you are growing me, even in the small and ordinary moments. Teach me to celebrate each step forward with gratitude. When I start striving for perfection, gently pull me back to Your grace and remind me that You are shaping me day by day. Amen.

Challenge of the Week:

Write down one way you've grown since becoming a mom spiritually, emotionally, or even in a simple daily routine. Thank God for that growth, and ask Him to continue shaping you with patience and love.

Mom Tip of the Week:

At the end of each day, instead of focusing on what you didn't finish, name three things you did with love. Progress is built through small, grace-filled moments, not perfect ones.

Trusting God's Timing

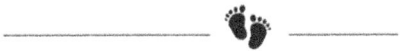

"He has made everything beautiful in its time."
-Ecclesiastes 3:11

Motherhood has a way of stretching your patience in ways you never expected. You wait for naps that don't happen... for routines that won't stick... for milestones that seem to take forever. It's completely natural to want things to fall into place quickly, especially when you're tired and doing your best every day. But the truth is, God's timing rarely matches ours, and yet, His timing is always right.

There are days when waiting feels frustrating, even discouraging. Maybe you're longing for a full night of sleep or hoping for your baby to finally settle into a rhythm. Maybe you're waiting for your own body to heal or for your emotions to find steady ground again. These waiting seasons can feel like detours, but in God's hands, they become sacred spaces where He gently invites you to trust Him more.

When we try to rush what God is still forming, we miss the beauty in the process. Just as your baby grows at exactly the pace they're meant to, God is working in you at the pace *He* knows you need. Your waiting is not wasted, it's shaping you. Teaching you to rest. Teaching you to depend on Him. Teaching you to believe that He is working, even when you can't see how.

Some of the deepest growth happens in the slow, ordinary days, the quiet mornings, the long nights, the moments that feel repetitive or unnoticed. These are the places where faith takes root.

So, when things don't happen as quickly as you hoped, remind yourself of this: God is never late. He knows you. He knows your child. And He knows exactly when each season should begin and end. The timing He chooses will always be more beautiful than the plan you would have created on your own.

Prayer:

Lord, help me trust Your timing, especially when patience feels hard. When I'm tempted to rush ahead or worry about what's next, remind me that You are working all things together for my good. Teach me to rest in Your pace and find peace in the waiting. Amen.

Challenge of the Week:
When something doesn't go the way you planned, pause instead of reacting. Take a slow breath and whisper: "God, I trust Your timing." Let those words settle your heart.

Mom Tip of the Week:
Avoid comparing your baby's progress or your own journey with anyone else's. Every child grows at their own rhythm, and every mother does too. Trust the pace God has set for your family.

Julie Whitecotton

Grace for Today

"My grace is sufficient for you, for My power is made perfect in weakness."
- 2 Corinthians 12:9

Some days in motherhood feel like a gift when your baby naps well, the house is quiet for a moment, and you catch yourself thinking, *I can do this.* Other days... well, everything seems to fall apart before you've even had a chance to drink your coffee. The baby is fussy, the chores pile up, and your emotions feel stretched thin. On those days, it's easy to focus on where you feel you failed or what you didn't get right.

But God never asks you to measure your worth by your perfection. He asks you to rely on Him.

His grace isn't just enough for your smooth, peaceful days, it's especially enough for the messy, exhausting, tear-filled ones. When you feel weak, when you're overwhelmed, when you feel like you're barely holding it together, that's not the end of your strength... It's the beginning of *His*.

Weakness doesn't mean you've failed as a mom. It means you're human. And it's often in those very moments when you feel empty or unsure that God's presence becomes the most real. He meets you in the laundry pile. He meets you in the dark during midnight feedings. He meets you in the quiet tears you wipe away before anyone notices. His grace gently covers the parts of you that feel tired, uncertain, or imperfect.

Permit yourself to rest in that grace. You don't need tomorrow's strength today. God gives grace in daily portions enough for this hour, this moment, this breath. And when tomorrow comes, His mercy will meet you all over again.

Your job isn't to be perfect. It's to lean on the One who is.

Prayer:

Lord, thank You for the gift of Your grace, steady, unending, and always enough. When I feel weak or overwhelmed, remind me that Your strength fills the places I cannot. Help me release the pressure to do it all, and teach me to rely on You for what I need today. Amen.

Challenge of the Week:

Each morning, pause and pray: "Lord, give me the grace I need for today, no more, no less." Notice how He provides exactly what your day requires.

Mom Tip of the Week:

Don't drag yesterday's guilt or tomorrow's worries into today. Take motherhood one day, even one hour at a time. God's grace meets you right here, in the present, not in perfection.

Peace in the Chaos

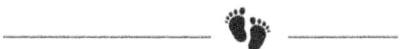

"The Lord gives strength to His people; the Lord blesses His people with peace."
- Psalm 29:11

Motherhood is this tender, unpredictable blend of joy and chaos. One moment, your baby is snuggled against you and everything feels soft and sweet... and the next moment, there's a spill, a cry, or a to-do list that's somehow longer than it was five minutes ago. It's easy to think peace is something you'll experience *later* when life slows down, when the house is quiet, when the baby finally sleeps through the night.

But God's peace isn't something you have to wait for. It's something He offers you right now, even in the thick of the mess.
True peace doesn't come from having a perfectly calm environment. It comes from having a heart anchored in God's presence. He never promised to remove every challenge, but He *did* promise to be with you in each one. And that makes all the difference.

When you invite Him into your everyday moments, the loud ones, the stressful ones, the ordinary ones, He brings a kind of stillness the world cannot touch. Each time you choose patience instead of panic... a whispered prayer instead of frustration... a deep breath instead of spiraling thoughts... You are allowing His peace to steady your heart.

Yes, there will always be dishes. There will always be laundry. There will always be moments where things feel like "too much." But peace isn't found in perfection or quiet, it's found in remembering that God is right there with you, holding your heart steady even when everything else feels scattered.

So, when the chaos rises, pause, breathe. Remember: You carry peace within you because the Prince of Peace lives in you.

Prayer:

Lord, thank You for being my peace when everything around me feels chaotic. When my heart starts to race and my thoughts begin to swirl, teach me to pause and lean into Your presence. Calm my spirit, steady my mind, and remind me that I can rest in You no matter what my day looks like. Amen.

Challenge of the Week:

When your day starts to feel overwhelming, stop and take three slow, deep breaths. With each breath, quietly say: "The Lord is my peace." Let that truth settle into your heart.

Mom Tip of the Week:

Create small pockets of calm throughout your day: light a candle, play soft worship music, or step outside for a few minutes of fresh air. Even tiny moments of stillness can help your heart stay rooted in God's peace.

Julie Whitecotton

Anchored in Hope

"We have this hope as an anchor for the soul, firm and secure."
-Hebrews 6:19

    Motherhood can feel like riding waves of love, joy, fear, exhaustion, gratitude, and uncertainty all at the same time. Some days you feel steady, like you've finally found your footing. Other days, even the smallest thing can knock you off balance, and you find yourself wondering if you're doing any of this right.

    In those moments, it's easy to lose perspective. But God offers you something solid, something unmoving hope.

    This hope isn't fragile, temporary, or dependent on perfect circumstances. It is strong. Steady. Secure. The kind of hope that holds you when you feel overwhelmed and reminds you that God is still writing your story, even when your days feel long and your emotions feel scattered.

    There will be seasons when things unfold more slowly than you expected, when milestones take time, when healing doesn't happen as quickly as you prayed for, or when you feel stuck in a routine that seems endless. But hope whispers, *"This won't last forever."* The long nights will eventually ease. Strength will return. Joy will rise again.

And God, who has carried you this far, will continue to carry you through.

Anchoring your heart in hope doesn't mean pretending everything is okay. It means trusting that God is at work even when you can't see what He's doing. It means believing His promises are still true on the days when your emotions feel shaky. You may not see the full picture right now, but the Artist does, and His hands are steady.

When you cling to hope, you're really clinging to Him, the God who never changes, never leaves, and never lets go of you or your child.

Julie Whitecotton

Prayer:

Lord, thank You for being my anchor when life feels uncertain. When doubt or fear begins to tug at my heart, remind me of the unshakable hope I have in You. Help me trust Your promises even when I can't see the full picture. Strengthen my heart and steady my spirit with Your faithfulness. Amen.

Challenge of the Week:

Each morning, take a moment to write down or speak out loud one thing you're hopeful for, big or small. Let hope become part of your daily rhythm, gently shifting your focus toward God's goodness.

Mom Tip of the Week:

Start a simple "hope jar." Each time you experience a blessing, a sweet moment, a small victory, an unexpected encouragement, write it on a slip of paper. On the hard days, open the jar and remind yourself of the many ways God has already shown up.

Strong Foundations

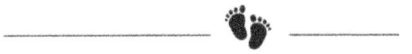

"Therefore, everyone who hears these words of mine and puts them into practice is like a wise man who built his house on the rock."
-Matthew 7:24

Every mother dream of giving her child a strong start, a home filled with love, stability, and a faith that can carry them through life. But when you're in the middle of sleepless nights, unpredictable days, and endless responsibilities, the idea of "building a strong foundation" can feel intimidating. You may worry about doing everything right, teaching the right things, or being the perfect example.

But here's the beautiful truth: The best foundation you can give your child doesn't come from perfect parenting, it comes from your relationship with God.

When your life is settled on His Word, your home naturally becomes a place where peace, patience, and grace take root. Your baby may not understand your prayers or the Scriptures you read, but they will feel the calm that comes from a mom who draws her strength from Christ.

Julie Whitecotton

Picture your faith as the solid rock beneath your family. Storms will come, rough nights, unexpected challenges, moments where you feel worn thin. But if your heart is anchored in Jesus, you will not be shaken. Every quiet prayer you whisper over your baby, every time you choose gentleness over frustration, every verse you hold onto when you feel overwhelmed, each of these becomes part of the foundation God is helping you build.

You may not see the structure rising yet, but brick by brick, day by day, something eternal is forming.

God isn't asking you to be flawless; He's simply asking you to stay close to Him. As you grow in His love, your child will see it in your patience, in your forgiveness, in the peace that fills your home. You're showing them what it means to build a life on the Rock that never crumbles.

Prayer:

Lord, help me build my home on You. Let Your truth steady my heart and shape the way I speak, respond, and love. Teach me to build with grace, patience, and faith, knowing that every small act of love is planting something eternal in my child's life. Amen.

Challenge of the Week:
Choose one Scripture to speak over your family throughout the week. Write it on your mirror, tuck it into your Bible, or place it somewhere you'll see often. Let God's promises be the foundation your home stands on.

Mom Tip of the Week:
Create simple, peaceful rhythms for your home, soft worship music in the morning, a short prayer before meals, or a gentle blessing at bedtime. These little moments become spiritual bricks that help build a strong, lasting foundation of faith.

Julie Whitecotton

Wisdom in Waiting

"If any of you lacks wisdom, you should ask God, who gives generously to all without finding fault, and it will be given to you."
- James 1:5

Motherhood is a journey filled with countless decisions, when to feed, how to soothe, whether to wake the baby or let them sleep, and how to care for yourself while caring for your child. Some days you feel confident, and other days you question if you're doing any of it right. It's normal to feel unsure; motherhood is holy work, but it's not simple work.

Here's the comforting truth: God never meant for you to figure everything out alone.

His Word promises that when you ask Him for wisdom, He gives it freely, not with frustration, not with judgment, but with generosity and love. He doesn't shake His head at your questions or your uncertainty. He delights in guiding you.

Wisdom doesn't always come as a lightning bolt or a clear voice. Often it shows up as a quiet calm in your heart... a gentle pause before reacting... an inner nudge that helps you see your baby's needs, or your own, a little more clearly. God's wisdom helps you know when to speak and when to stay silent, when to rest and when to push through, when to let something go and when to hold it close.

Learning to walk in God's wisdom often means learning to wait. There will be moments when the answers don't come right away. But waiting doesn't mean God is ignoring you. He's preparing you. He's teaching you how to listen for His voice, even in the middle of busy days and noisy moments.

And the beautiful thing is this: every time you bring Him your questions, even though small, imperfect prayers, you're building a rhythm of doing motherhood hand-in-hand with Him. Wisdom grows in that relationship... one day, one prayer, one decision at a time.

Prayer:

Lord, I need Your wisdom today and every day. When I feel unsure or overwhelmed, help me slow down and listen for Your voice. Thank you for giving wisdom generously and patiently. Guide my steps, shape my choices, and help me walk in Your truth with a peaceful heart. Amen.

Challenge of the Week:
Before making any decision, big or small, pause and pray: "Lord, give me wisdom and peace." Then trust the direction that settles your spirit instead of stirring it.

Mom Tip of the Week:
Keep a small notebook or the notes app on your phone nearby. Jot down prayers, insights, or moments when you feel God giving you clarity. On hard days, those reminders will show you just how faithfully He speaks.

Walking by Faith

"For we walk by faith, not by sight."
- 2 Corinthians 5:7

    Motherhood is, in so many ways, an act of pure faith. Every day you wake up and step into the unknown, guessing, learning, trying again, and praying that what you're doing is enough. So much of what matters most happens where you can't see it: the quiet growth happening inside your baby, the strengthening happening inside your heart, the gentle work God is doing behind the scenes in your family.

    It's natural to long for visible signs that things are working: more sleep, a calm routine, a feeling of control. But the path of faith doesn't always give us instant results. Instead, it invites us to trust that God is moving, even when our eyes can't see the outcome.

    Walking by faith means believing that your small, unseen acts of love are shaping something beautiful. It means trusting that the prayers whispered in the dark, the sacrifices no one else notices, and the patience you choose when you feel empty, all of it is sowing seeds that will grow in time. You may not see the fruit yet, but Jesus sees every step you take.

It also means letting go of the pressure to control everything. Faith isn't about having a perfect plan; it's about holding onto the One who knows the way. God doesn't hand you a map He offers His hand. And when you take each step with Him, you'll find that even the winding, confusing paths lead you toward peace.

So today, don't worry about seeing the whole journey. Just take the next step, trusting that God is walking it with you. He's guiding you, holding you, and growing you through every moment, even the ones that feel ordinary or uncertain.

Prayer:

Lord, teach me to walk by faith, especially in the moments when I can't see what's ahead. Help me trust Your leading and rest in the truth that You are working even when I don't understand. Strengthen my heart and steady my steps as I follow You, one day at a time. Amen.

Challenge of the Week:

Think of one area where you've been struggling to trust God. Write it down and pray: **"Lord, I choose faith over fear."** Then take one small, practical step forward as an act of trust.

Mom Tip of the Week:

Don't rush the journey. Faith grows in small, steady steps. Celebrate the quiet victories, the moments of patience, the tiny breakthroughs, the prayers you remembered to pray. These are signs that God is lovingly guiding your path.

Julie Whitecotton

Compassion in Motion

————————  ————————

*"Be kind and compassionate to one another,
forgiving each other, just as in
Christ God forgave you."*
- Ephesians 4:32

Motherhood has a way of softening and reshaping the heart. The love you feel for your little one is fierce, protective, and unconditional... but it also pulls out parts of you that you never knew were there humility, tenderness, and a depth of compassion that only grows with time.

But let's be honest: the constant needs, the interrupted sleep, and the emotional weight of caring for a tiny human can make kindness feel harder some days. Not just kindness to others... but kindness to yourself. It's so easy to snap, to feel guilty, or to be your own harshest critic.

That's why compassion isn't just something you *feel*, it's something you choose. It is love set in motion.
It's the soft word you offer when irritation rises. It's choosing understanding over frustration. It's the moment you forgive quickly instead of letting bitterness take root. It's the gentle way you comfort your baby, even when you're exhausted.

And here's the powerful thing: your baby absorbs every bit of it. Long before they can speak, they are learning what love looks like by watching you. The compassion you show in small moments becomes the soil where kindness and empathy will grow in their heart.

But compassion must also begin with *you*. God never intended for you to mother from an empty place. The same grace He pours over your life each morning is meant to restore you, steady you, and remind you that you are deeply loved. When you fall short, He doesn't pull away. He draws near.

Let His compassion toward you become the compassion that flows through you into your home, your relationships, and your own weary heart.

Prayer:

Lord, thank You for loving me with endless compassion. Teach me to show that same kindness in my home, in my words, my actions, and the way I respond when I'm tired or overwhelmed. Help me forgive quickly and love deeply. And when I feel empty, fill me again with Your mercy. Amen.

Challenge of the Week:

Each day this week, look for one simple way to show compassion to your partner, a friend, another mom, or even a stranger. Kindness in motion creates ripples of grace.

Mom Tip of the Week:

Practice speaking to yourself the way you speak to your child, gently, patiently, and with encouragement. The compassion you show yourself becomes the compassion you're able to offer others.

The Beauty of Patience

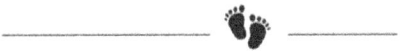

"Be completely humble and gentle; be patient, bearing with one another in love."
- Ephesians 4:2

Patience might be one of the hardest lessons a mother learns. Every part of motherhood invites you into some form of waiting, waiting for your baby to settle, waiting for sleep to come, waiting for routines to form, waiting for milestones to unfold. Some days, the waiting feels endless, and you may catch yourself wishing everything would move a little faster, or feel a little easier.

But motherhood has a way of slowing life down and teaching you to breathe differently. These moments of delay and interruption aren't wasted; they are shaping you. They are strengthening parts of your heart you never knew needed strengthening. And through it all, God is gently whispering, *"Trust My timing."*

True patience isn't passive. It's not simply gritting your teeth and enduring. It's an active choice choosing to respond with love instead of frustration, choosing to breathe instead of snap, choosing to trust instead of rush. Each time you pause in a moment of tension, you are teaching your heart and your little one what love looks like under pressure.

Patience is one of the most beautiful gifts you can offer your home. It turns chaos into calm. It softens your voice. It brings peace into places that once felt overwhelming. And slowly, you begin to notice: the situations that once made you anxious now invite you to practice grace.

Patience is love waiting with a peaceful heart. And every time you choose compassion over irritation, every time you take a deep breath instead of reacting, heaven takes notice. God is using this season to cultivate gentleness within you, forming the fruit of patience one choice, one moment, one prayer at a time.

You may not always *feel* patient, and that's okay. The Holy Spirit is at work in you, growing what you cannot grow on your own.

Prayer:

Lord, thank You for the lessons woven into this season of waiting. When impatience rises or I feel overwhelmed, remind me of how patient You are with me. Help me slow down, breathe deeply, and choose love over frustration. Grow within me a quiet strength that reflects Your peace. Amen.

Challenge of the Week:

Each time impatience begins to rise, stop for just a moment and whisper: "Lord, give me Your peace." Let every stressful moment become a doorway to prayer.

Mom Tip of the Week:

Remember, your child learns patience by watching you. The calm in your tone and the gentleness in your reactions teach more than any lesson. Gentle hearts build gentle homes.

Julie Whitecotton

Joy in Service

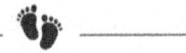

"Serve one another humbly in love."
- Galatians 5:13

Motherhood is a beautiful calling, but it is also one of the most demanding forms of service you will ever offer. You serve when you rock your baby long after your arms are tired... when you get up in the night, even though you barely slept... when you put aside your own comfort to meet the needs of someone who depends on you completely.

These acts of love often happen quietly, without applause or recognition. But God sees them all. And in His eyes, every small act of service, every diaper changed, every meal prepared, every tear wiped away holds eternal weight.

Jesus showed us what joyful service looks like. He didn't serve out of duty but out of deep, generous love. When you serve your family with that same heart, even in your exhaustion, you're reflecting Him. The work may feel ordinary, but it is holy. These daily tasks that seem repetitive or unseen are actually shaping your home and your heart.

Here's something important to remember: Joyful service doesn't mean ignoring your own needs. It means allowing God to fill you so you can pour out from a place of strength, not depletion. When you nourish your spirit through prayer, Scripture, and rest, your service becomes worship, not burden. A mom connected to God's presence brings peace into every corner of her home. Your service is not wasted. It is not unnoticed. It is love in action, and heaven honors it.

Prayer:

Lord, thank You for the privilege of serving my family. When I feel tired or unseen, remind me that You notice every act of love. Help me serve with a joyful heart, one that reflects Your kindness and compassion. Let my home be filled with Your love through every simple task I do. Amen.

Challenge of the Week:

Pick one chore that usually feels draining or frustrating. As you do it, whisper a simple prayer: **"Lord, I offer this to You."** Let that moment become an act of worship instead of a burden.

Mom Tip of the Week:

You can't pour out joy if you're running on empty. Make space each day for a small moment that refreshes you: a quiet prayer, a cup of tea, a few deep breaths. Filling your cup helps you serve with love.

Faith Over Fear

"When I am afraid, I put my trust in You."
- Psalm 56:3

Motherhood brings a kind of love that is powerful and protective, the kind that makes you hold your baby a little closer and pray over them a little harder. But with that deep love often comes fear. Fear over their health. Fear over their future. Fear that you won't always know what to do or how to do it "right." These worries can slip into your heart quietly and begin to weigh heavily on your mind.
But God gently reminds you: fear was never meant to lead your life, faith was.

Fear focuses on everything that *might* happen. Faith focuses on the God who already knows, sees, and holds every moment.

There is a simple yet powerful truth woven through Scripture: Fear and faith cannot fill the same space. One always pushes out the other.

Feeling anxious doesn't mean you're failing; it means you have another chance to choose trust. Faith doesn't erase fear instantly, and it doesn't make every worry disappear. But faith gives you the strength to keep moving even when you feel afraid. It lets you breathe again. It reminds you that God is holding both you and your child fully, gently, and securely.

Think of all the ways God has been faithful in your life so far. All the prayers He has answered, all the moments He carried you, all the times He came through when you didn't see a way. That same faithfulness covers this season, too.

When fear starts whispering "what if," speak the name of Jesus and let His peace interrupt the worry. Fear may knock at your door, but it doesn't get to stay. Faith opens the door and invites peace in.

Prayer:

Lord, when fear rises in my heart, draw me back to You. Remind me that You are near, that You see every detail, and that nothing is outside Your control. Replace my anxious thoughts with Your peace, and strengthen my faith until trust becomes my first response. Amen.

Challenge of the Week:
Whenever fear shows up, even for a moment, pause and speak out loud: "God, I trust You." Let those words interrupt the fear every single time.

Mom Tip of the Week:
Pay attention to what feeds your fears: constant scrolling, comparison, or overwhelming information. Protect your peace. Choose Scripture, prayer, and truth instead. Faith grows strongest when fear is starved.

Julie Whitecotton

Love That Never Fails

————  ————

"Love never fails."
-1 Corinthians 13:8

Every single day, without even realizing it, you live out love in the most practical and sacrificial ways. You show love in the middle of the night when you drag yourself out of bed to soothe your baby. You show love when you offer early-morning snuggles even though you're still exhausted. You show love in the countless quiet tasks of feeding, rocking, washing, and comforting that no one sees but God.

This kind of love isn't loud or glamorous.

It's steady.

It's patient.

It's persistent.

It's the kind of love that keeps giving even when you're running on empty.

And this love, the love you're learning as a mother, is the closest reflection of God's heart. His love never quits, never runs out, never gives up. Through motherhood, you're growing to love in a way that mirrors His own unfailing love.

But let's be honest... loving like this isn't always easy. Some days you feel stretched thin, and your patience feels fragile. Some days, you wonder if you're doing enough or if your love is even making a difference. On those days, remember this:

Love is not measured by perfection. Love is measured by faithfulness.

God sees every unseen act of love, every tear you wipe away, every moment you choose gentleness when frustration rises, every sacrifice you make without a second thought. Your love matters because it plants seeds of security and grace deep within your child's heart.

And when you feel like you've reached your limit, don't forget: You were never meant to love in your own strength. God's unfailing love is the well you draw from the strength that carries you, the peace that steadies you, the grace that fills the cracks.

You're not just caring for your child; you are showing them what God's love looks like through the tenderness of your actions. And that kind of love? It will never fail.

Julie Whitecotton

Prayer:

Lord, thank You for Your love that never runs dry. Teach me to love with Your patience, Your kindness, and Your grace, especially on the days when I feel weary or overwhelmed. Fill my heart with Your Spirit so that every act of care becomes an offering of love that honors You. Amen.

Challenge of the Week:

Take a few minutes to write a note or prayer for your child, something simple, something from your heart, reminding them how deeply they are loved by both you and the God who created them.

Mom Tip of the Week:

When frustration starts to rise, pause and whisper: "Love never fails." This gentle reminder can soften your heart and help you respond with grace instead of pressure.

Strength in Surrender

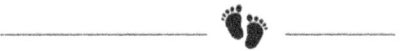

"The Lord will fight for you; you need only to be still."
- Exodus 14:14

Motherhood often feels like you're juggling a dozen things at once, trying to keep your home running, trying to meet every need, trying to stay patient, trying to look strong even when you're exhausted inside. And no matter how capable or organized you are, there inevitably comes a moment when you realize something important:

You can't control everything. And that moment, though humbling, is actually holy. Because that's where surrender begins.

Surrender isn't about giving up or failing. It's about handing over the weight you were never meant to carry your fears, your plans, your exhaustion, to the God who never tires, never falters, and never stops fighting for you.

Think of Moses standing in front of the Red Sea, trapped between danger and the unknown. God didn't tell him to try harder or think faster. God said something beautifully simple: "Be still."

Julie Whitecotton

That same whisper is spoken over your heart today. When your mind spirals with "what ifs," When your heart beats fast with the pressure to do everything right, when fear tells you you're alone
God leans close and says, "Be still, My daughter. I am fighting for you."

Surrender requires a different kind of strength, not the strength that pushes through, but the strength that lets go. The kind that says: "Lord, I trust You more than I trust my own understanding." And as you practice surrender, something beautiful happens.

>Your load lightens.

>Your thoughts are quiet.

>Your spirit finds rest again.

You begin to realize that surrender is not weakness, it is freedom. It makes space for God's power to steady you, guide you, and work through you in ways you couldn't on your own.

You don't have to hold everything together. He already is.

Prayer:

Lord, teach me the strength of surrender. When I try to carry everything in my own power, remind me that You are already fighting for me. Help me release my worries, rest in Your promises, and trust that You are guiding my family with love and wisdom. Amen.

Challenge of the Week:
Each day, choose one worry you've been holding onto. Speak it out loud and say: "God, I release this to You." Let surrender become a gentle daily habit.

Mom Tip of the Week:
You don't have to do everything perfectly to be a loving, present, incredible mom. Let go of the pressure to control every detail. Focus on connection, not perfection. Your baby needs your heart more than your flawless performance.

Finding Beauty in the Ordinary

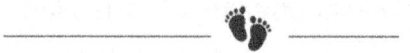

"Whatever you do, do it all for the glory of God."
-1 Corinthians 10:31

So much of motherhood happens in the quiet, repetitive moments, the feedings that feel endless, the diaper changes that seem constant, the laundry that never really stops. Days can blend, and it's easy to feel like you're just going through motions without seeing much progress.

But here's the truth: God sees beauty where the world only sees routine.

Every diaper you change, every tear you wipe, every gentle word you speak when you're bone-tired, these aren't small things. They are expressions of love. They are reflections of God's heart. And in His eyes, they matter deeply.

It's easy to imagine that glorifying God means doing big, bold, public things, leading ministries, going on mission trips, and standing on stages. But for many mothers, the most sacred ministry happens quietly at home. Your kitchen becomes a sanctuary. Your rocking chair becomes a place of prayer. Your whispered lullabies become worship.

Heaven sees what no one else does. God treasures the love you pour into the ordinary because love is never ordinary to Him.

And when you feel weary or invisible in the routine, remember this: God is present in it all. He is in the soft rhythm of your day, in the hum of simple tasks, in the warmth of your home. He's not waiting for you to do something "big." He's honoring the faithfulness you show in the small things.

You're not just checking off tasks. You are building a foundation of security, peace, and love for your child. You are participating in holy work, moment by moment.

And when your heart turns toward Him, even the simplest tasks shine with divine purpose.

Prayer:

Lord, thank You for being with me in every part of my day, even in the ordinary moments' others might overlook. Help me see the beauty You place in the simple rhythms of motherhood. Let every act of care, no matter how small, reflect Your love and bring glory to Your name. Amen.

Challenge of the Week:
Choose one routine task, feeding, rocking, folding laundry, or even washing dishes, and turn it into worship. Whisper a prayer of gratitude as you do it, and invite God into that moment.

Mom Tip of the Week:
Anchor your perspective in gratitude when you remember *why* you're doing these everyday tasks, even the ordinary ones, and start to feel extraordinary.

God's Faithfulness Never Fails

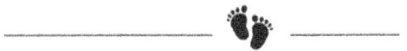

"The steadfast love of the Lord never ceases; His mercies never come to an end; they are new every morning; great is Your faithfulness."
- Lamentations 3:22–23

Every morning ushers in a new piece of your motherhood story. Some mornings you wake up hopeful and strong, ready to face a fresh day. Other mornings, you open your eyes already weary, wondering how you'll make it through the next set of needs, tasks, or emotions. But whether you rise with joy or with heaviness, one thing remains unshaken: God's faithfulness meets you there.

He is just as present in the long, sleepless nights as He is in the peaceful ones. His love doesn't depend on how put-together you feel or how smoothly your day begins. His mercy doesn't hinge on your performance as a mom. It's new every morning simply because you are His.

There will be days when you question yourself, moments when you wonder if you're doing enough, loving enough, or handling things the "right" way. But God's faithfulness gently covers those doubts with grace. He isn't asking you to be perfect; He's inviting you to trust Him.

His mercy follows you into every corner of your day, into the dishes in the sink, the diapers that need changing, the whispered prayers you speak over your baby. Each sunrise is His personal reminder that yesterday's struggles are behind you and today is another chance to rest in His love.

When you feel weary, pause and look back. Think of how far God has already carried you. Through pregnancy. Through birth. Through nights you thought you couldn't survive. Through fears you never voiced. Through emotions you didn't expect. He has been faithful every step of the way.

And He hasn't changed, not now, not ever. His love doesn't run out. His mercy doesn't expire. His strength never weakens. Take heart, mama. The God who carried you this far will continue to carry you and your child. His faithfulness never fails.

Prayer:

Lord, thank You for Your steady, unchanging faithfulness. On the days I feel worn down or uncertain, remind me that Your mercy is new and Your love is constant. Help me rest in the truth that You will never leave me, and You will never fail me. Amen.

Challenge of the Week:

Each morning, before you reach for your phone or start your routine, speak these words out loud: "Your mercies are new today." Let that truth reset your heart before the day begins.

Mom Tip of the Week:

Begin a simple "faithfulness journal." Write down answered prayers, moments of unexpected peace, or blessings throughout the week. Pull it out on hard days and let it remind you: God has been faithful before, and He will be faithful again.

The Gift of Gentleness

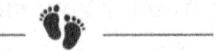

*"Let your gentleness be evident to all.
The Lord is near."*
- Philippians 4:5

Motherhood gives you countless opportunities to practice gentleness, often more than you ever imagined. There are moments when you handle your baby with such softness it makes your heart melt... and moments when you realize how quickly patience can slip away when you're tired, stretched thin, or overwhelmed.

But real gentleness doesn't come from trying harder or pretending to be calm. It grows out of *being close to God*.

When your heart rests in His presence, gentleness becomes something He produces in you like fruit growing quietly on a branch. His Spirit softens your reactions, strengthens your patience, and steadies your voice even when everything around you feels chaotic.

Gentleness isn't weakness. It is strength guided by love. It's the soft tone instead of the sharp one. It's the deep breath instead of the snap of anger. It's the tender word that soothes before frustration has a chance to spread.

When you respond gently, you are reflecting the heart of Jesus, the One who carried compassion wherever He went, even into messy, demanding situations. Your baby may not remember the details of these early days, but they *will* grow up feeling the warmth and peace that flows from a gentle mother.

And gentleness isn't just something you give to others, it's something you must give to yourself. Be gentle with yourself as you learn. Be gentle when you make mistakes. Be gentle when you feel like you're falling short.

God isn't watching you with disappointment. He is walking beside you with kindness, understanding, and unfailing love.

The gentleness you show your child is the same gentleness He pours over you each morning. And as that truth sinks deeper into your heart, your home begins to feel more like His soft, steady, peaceful, and full of grace.

Prayer:

Lord, thank You for the gentleness You show me every day. Teach me to offer that same spirit to my child, my family, and myself. When I feel overwhelmed or frustrated, calm my heart and remind myself that You are near. Let my words and actions reflect Your peace and kindness. Amen.

Challenge of the Week:

When frustration starts to rise, pause before reacting. Whisper: "Lord, help me respond with gentleness." Watch how peace settles into the moment.

Mom Tip of the Week:

Try lowering your voice instead of raising it. A soft tone brings calm quicker than anything else to your child, and to your own heart. Gentleness grows every time you choose grace.

When You Feel Overwhelmed

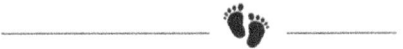

"When my heart is overwhelmed, lead me to the rock that is higher than I."
- Psalm 61:2

Some days as a mom can feel like waves crashing in faster than you can catch your breath. The needs don't stop, the decisions pile up, and your body and heart feel stretched in ways you never expected. You love your baby deeply, yet you can still feel drained, emotional, or unsure. And that doesn't make you a bad mother, it makes you human.

God sees those moments. He sees the tears you wipe before anyone notices. He sees the exhaustion you push through. He sees the weight you quietly carry. And He never intended for you to carry it alone.

David's words in this psalm sound a lot like the cry of a tired mother: *"Lord, I can't do this on my own. I need you."* And God responds with an invitation not to be stronger, not to push harder, but to *come closer*.

When you're overwhelmed, you don't have to fix everything. You need to look up.

Lift your eyes from the noise, the clutter, the "what ifs," and the pressure you put on yourself. Look to the Rock that is higher than your emotions, higher than your circumstances, higher than your fears. He is steady when everything around you feels shaky. He is strong when you feel weak. He is gentle when you're fragile.

Being overwhelmed doesn't mean you're failing; it means you're carrying more than you were designed to carry. God never asked you to be unbreakable; He asked you to be His. And in His presence, your heart finds rest, your mind finds clarity, and your spirit finds peace.

You are not alone in this season, not for one moment. God is your refuge, your strength, and your steady place to stand.

Prayer:

Lord, when my heart feels overwhelmed, draw me close to You. Be my strength when I feel weak and my peace when my mind is restless. Lift my eyes above the noise of my day and anchor me in Your love. Remind me that I don't walk this journey alone. You are my Rock, faithful and near. Amen.

Challenge of the Week:

When overwhelm rises, pause. Take one slow breath and say out loud: "God is my strength." Repeat it until your heart begins to settle and peace starts to return.

Mom Tip of the Week:

Permit yourself to simplify. Release the tasks that can wait. Focus on what matters most: rest, connection, and grace. Overwhelm fades when you choose peace over pressure.

Julie Whitecotton

God's Perfect Provision

"And my God will meet all your needs according to the riches of His glory in Christ Jesus."
-Philippians 4:19

Motherhood can bring a whole new set of worries, worries about finances, worries about sleep, worries about whether you can give enough of yourself emotionally, physically, and spiritually. You may find yourself wondering, *"Do I have enough? Am I enough?"* Those thoughts can weigh heavily on a mama's heart.

But here's the truth: God has never asked you to be the source, only to trust the Source.

His Word doesn't say He'll meet *some* of your needs or *most* of them. He promises to meet all of them not out of scarcity, but out of the overflowing riches of His glory. His supply is endless, even when yours runs thin.

Sometimes His provision shows up quietly, in ways you might overlook: a neighbor offering help, a baby who suddenly settles after a long cry, a moment of unexpected peace in the middle of a messy day. Other times, His provision looks like strength you didn't know you had or wisdom that comes just when you need it most. He provides in ways that are both miraculous and beautifully ordinary.

You're not walking through motherhood alone. The same God who fed thousands with a few loaves and fish, who provided manna in the wilderness, who cared for Elijah by sending a raven, that same God is caring for you.

Your home, your heart, and your family are not beyond His provision. Where you feel empty, He fills. Where you feel weak, He sustains. Where you feel stretched, He steps in.

You may not always see the answer right away, but you can trust that God's timing, though rarely early, is always perfect. And His care for you is personal, tender, and complete.

Prayer:

Father, thank You for being my faithful provider. When worry rises in my heart, remind me of all the ways You've already taken care of me. Teach me to rest in Your abundance instead of striving in my own strength. I trust You to meet every need for me, for my child, and for our home. Amen.

Challenge of the Week:

Start a simple "provision list" this week. Write down each small way God provides a moment of peace, a helping hand, an answered prayer. Let your list become a reminder that He is faithful every single day.

Mom Tip of the Week:

When worries begin to swirl, speak this truth out loud: "God will provide." Let your own voice remind your heart to choose faith over fear.

Holding Onto Peace

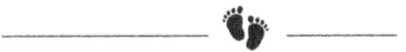

"Peace I leave with you; My peace I give you. I do not give to you as the world gives. Do not let your hearts be troubled and do not be afraid."
- John 14:27

Peace can feel like one of the hardest things to hold onto as a mom. When you think you've found a rhythm, something shifts: a cry from the other room, a sudden mess, a need that pulls you away from your plans. Motherhood is full of these interruptions, and they can make peace feel like something far out of reach.

But Jesus offers a kind of peace that isn't tied to silence, schedules, or perfect days. His peace isn't the kind the world gives, fragile, temporary, and easily disturbed. His peace is steady, deep, and rooted in His presence. It stays with you in the noise, in the piles of laundry, in the moments when you feel pulled in ten different directions.

This peace grows through small, intentional choices:

    Choosing prayer over panic.

    Choosing a deep breath over a quick reaction.

    Choosing gratitude over grumbling.

You won't get it perfect every time, no one does. But peace isn't about perfection; it's about returning to Him again and again. Jesus doesn't ask you to eliminate the chaos... just to let Him be your calm within it.

When your thoughts start to race or your patience starts slipping, pause. Close your eyes for a moment if you can. Whisper His name, *Jesus*. Let that simple act draw your heart back to Him. Peace isn't something you chase... It's something you receive. And it's already yours because He promised it.

You can face whatever today brings because you're not walking into it alone. His peace goes with you, surrounds you, and settles you even in the wildest moments of motherhood.

Prayer:

Lord, thank You for the peace that only comes from You. When my heart feels overwhelmed or anxious, draw me back into Your presence. Calm my thoughts. Steady my emotions. Let Your peace fill the atmosphere of my home and quiet the places in me that feel troubled. Amen.

Challenge of the Week:

Give yourself just a few quiet minutes each morning, even five, to breathe deeply, pray, and invite God's peace into your day before the noise begins.

Mom Tip of the Week:

Keep a short "peace verse" nearby, written on a sticky note, saved on your phone, or taped to your mirror. When frustration rises, speak it out loud. Scripture has a way of settling the heart in seconds.

Julie Whitecotton

Finding Balance in a Busy Season

———————— 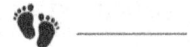 ————————

"There is a time for everything, and a season for every activity under the heavens."
- Ecclesiastes 3:1

Motherhood can feel like you're trying to juggle a dozen things while still holding a baby on your hip. There are days when you're torn between caring for your little one, managing your home, nurturing your relationships, and maybe keeping up with work. It's a lot. And in the middle of it all, you might catch yourself wondering, *How am I supposed to balance all of this without falling apart?*

Here's the truth: balance doesn't mean doing everything perfectly at the same time. It doesn't mean keeping every room spotless, every task completed, or every expectation met. Real balance begins when you recognize that this season of your life has its own unique rhythm, a rhythm God handpicked just for you.

This season is different from any other you've lived... and that's okay. It's slower in some ways, fuller in others, and more tender than words can express. God isn't asking you to be superwoman. He's not expecting you to keep every plate spinning. He's inviting you to lean into what matters most right now: your relationship with Him, your connection with your baby, and your own emotional and spiritual well-being.

Some things will go undone: dishes, messages, tasks you meant to finish. Let grace make peace with that. Balance isn't about doing everything... It's about doing the right things for *this* season. When you say "yes" to what brings peace and "no" to what steals it, you create space for God to strengthen and steady you.

Even Jesus stepped away from crowds to rest, breathe, and pray. If rest was important for Him, it's more than okay for you. Let God lead you into a gentle rhythm of grace, not rushed, not pressured, but steady and life-giving. He will help you find balance not by adding more to your days, but by helping you rely more deeply on Him.

Prayer:

Lord, help me find balance in this busy season. Show me what truly matters today, and give me the courage to let go of what doesn't. Teach me to rest in Your grace and trust Your leading as I care for my family and myself. Steady my heart, quiet my mind, and guide me gently through each moment. Amen.

Challenge of the Week:
Before the day begins, pause and ask God, "What matters most today?" Write down just one or two things He places on your heart and focus your energy there instead of trying to tackle everything.

Mom Tip of the Week:
Permit yourself to simplify. Pick one area: meals, chores, errands, or commitments, and intentionally make it easier. Balance grows when you create breathing room for peace.

The Blessing of Community

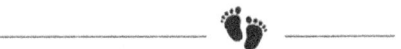

"Therefore, encourage one another and build each other up, just as in fact you are doing."
-1 Thessalonians 5:11

Motherhood was never designed to be walked alone. Yes, your love for your baby is powerful and beautiful, the kind of love that makes you want to do everything yourself. But even the strongest, most devoted mothers need help, support, and voices that remind them they're not alone. God gave us the gift of community because He knew we would need people to lean on, to laugh with, to pray with, and to hold us up on the days we feel like we're barely holding ourselves.

But reaching out isn't always easy. Maybe you worry about looking like you're struggling. Maybe you've been disappointed before. Maybe you're too tired to initiate a conversation. Whatever the reason, know this: community isn't built on perfection, it's built on honesty. Real connection happens when we drop the mask and allow others to see not only the highlights but also the hard parts.

Julie Whitecotton

The truth is, God often answers prayers through people. A friend who texts you right when you're overwhelmed. Another mom who says, "Me too," and suddenly you feel understood.

A warm meal was dropped off at your door. A kind word that reminds you that you're doing a better job than you think. These are not coincidences; they're God's gentle reminders that He sees you.

You don't have to carry the full weight of motherhood by yourself. Surround yourself with women who love Jesus and understand this season, women who will pray with you, speak life into you, and remind you of God's goodness when your own heart feels stretched thin. When you give and receive support, you're walking in the very design God created: a life woven together with others, strengthened through community, anchored in love.

Prayer:

Lord, thank You for the people You've placed around me. Help me to let others in instead of trying to carry everything alone. Teach me to be honest, open, and willing to give and receive support. Let my friendships be full of encouragement, grace, and Your love. Amen.

Challenge of the Week:

Reach out to one other mom this week, even with something simple like a message, a quick voice note, or sharing a cup of coffee. You never know how deeply that small connection might bless both of you.

Mom Tip of the Week:

Community grows through consistency, not perfection. Keep showing up even when you feel tired or messy because your presence may be the encouragement someone else has been praying for.

Julie Whitecotton

Blessed Beyond Measure

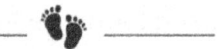

"Now to Him who can do immeasurably more than all we ask or imagine, according to His power that is at work within us."
- Ephesians 3:20

When you pause long enough to really look around, even in the middle of the dishes, the laundry piles, the late-night feedings, the toys scattered across the floor, you'll begin to see it: you are living in blessings you once prayed for.

It doesn't always feel magical. In fact, most blessings arrive dressed in ordinary clothes in the soft weight of your baby sleeping on your chest, in the tiny fingers wrapped around yours, in the sound of your child's laughter ringing through the house. These moments whisper reminders of a God who delights in giving more than you ever thought to ask for.

But blessings aren't always easy. Sometimes they come disguised as challenges that stretch your patience, test your strength, and remind you how much you need Jesus. Motherhood has a way of taking you past your own limits, not to break you, but to show you the power of God at work within you. The days that leave you weary may actually be the days He's doing the deepest work in your heart.

And still you are blessed beyond measure. Not because everything is perfect, not because you feel joyful every moment. But because God is with you in it all.

The same God who formed your child with care is also forming you. As you choose gratitude over frustration, as you notice His goodness in the small things, your eyes begin to open to the abundance around you. His presence in your home, His strength in your weaknesses, His joy tucked inside the ordinary, *these* are the blessings that can never be counted.

Pause today and look again. You'll see that His goodness has been woven into every corner of your life.

Julie Whitecotton

Prayer:

Lord, thank You for the blessings You've placed in my life, both big and small. Help me to slow down and notice Your goodness in the middle of my everyday moments. When I feel tired or overwhelmed, remind me that Your power is at work in me and that I am blessed beyond measure. Amen.

Challenge of the Week:

Start or update a simple gratitude list. Each day, write down three blessings, no matter how small. At the end of the week, read them aloud as a prayer of thanksgiving.

Mom Tip of the Week:

Gratitude shifts everything. When frustration rises, pause and thank God for one thing about that moment, even if it's simply the privilege of being the one who gets to love your child.

Rest in His Grace

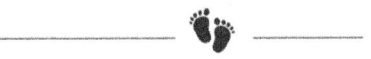

"Come to me, all you who are weary and burdened, and I will give you rest."
- Matthew 11:28

As a new mom, rest can feel like a foreign word, something you remember from another lifetime. There's always something calling your name: a cry from the crib, a bottle to wash, a task waiting on the counter. Even when you finally sit down, your mind might still be running through the next dozen things you need to do. And in the middle of all of this movement, Jesus whispers an invitation that feels almost too good to be true:

Come to Me... and I will give you rest. This rest He offers isn't only about sleep, though you could probably use more of that too. It's a deeper rest, a rest for your soul. It's the kind of rest that says, *You don't have to earn My love. You don't have to hold it all together. You are enough, even here... especially here.*

God's grace permits you to breathe. It gently quiets the voice that says you must do more, be more, or prove more. Grace says you can stop striving. You don't have to be a perfect mom to be a loved one.

Julie Whitecotton

Rest looks like pausing the pressure. Rest looks like saying "no" without guilt. Rest looks like receiving help without feeling weak. Rest looks like letting Jesus carry what was never meant to weigh you down.

And sometimes, rest is as simple as five slow breaths with your eyes closed, a moment of stillness where your heart can say, "Lord, I trust You." Because when you pause, even briefly, you're reminding your soul that God is the One holding everything together... not you.

He sees your weariness. He isn't disappointed in your exhaustion. He invites you closer, promising that His rest will meet you exactly where you are.

Prayer:

Lord, thank You for meeting me in my weariness with grace instead of pressure. Teach me how to rest in You, not just with my body, but with my heart. Help me release the weight I've been carrying and trust that You are holding me and my family together. Let Your peace settle over me today. Amen.

Challenge of the Week:

Each day, take a short break, even just a minute or two, to sit in quiet. No phone. No tasks. No guilt. Breathe deeply and thank God for His sustaining grace.

Mom Tip of the Week:

Rest doesn't have to be perfect or long to be meaningful. Maybe it's a nap, a quiet walk, a hot shower, or a peaceful minute with your eyes closed. However, it comes, receive it without apology. Rest is part of God's design for you.

Julie Whitecotton

Harvest of Blessings

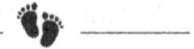

"Let us not become weary in doing good, for at the proper time we will reap a harvest if we do not give up."
- Galatians 6:9

Some seasons of motherhood feel like you're constantly sowing, giving, pouring out, and showing up day after day without seeing much come back. Your dry tears, repeat lessons, clean up messes, and steady your home with love... and sometimes you wonder, *Is any of this making a difference?*

But God sees every seed you plant, even the ones that feel small or unnoticed. Every time you choose patience instead of frustration, every time you pray over your child, even half-asleep in the middle of the night, every sacrifice you make out of sheer love is a seed He promises to water. Nothing given in love is ever wasted.

The truth is, much of motherhood happens beneath the surface. Growth doesn't always show up in immediate results. Just like a farmer can't see roots forming underground, you don't always see how God is shaping your child or shaping you. But He's working quietly, faithfully, perfectly in His timing.

There will be days when you feel weary, stretched thin, or unsure. On those days, hold onto this promise: the harvest *will* come. Not instantly, not always in the way you expect, but in God's perfect season. One day, you'll look back and see that those long nights, those whispered prayers, those "small" acts of love were actually the foundation of something beautiful and lasting.

Keep going, mama. Keep loving, keep praying, keep showing up. God is growing something in your home that will one day take your breath away.

Julie Whitecotton

Prayer:

Lord, thank You for seeing every seed I plant, even the ones the world overlooks. When I feel tired or discouraged, strengthen me with Your Spirit. Help me trust that You are working beneath the surface and that nothing done in love is ever wasted. Keep my heart faithful and hopeful as I wait for the harvest You have promised. Amen.

Challenge of the Week:
Notice one area where you've been faithfully sowing, even if results are still hidden. Thank God for the quiet, unseen work He's already doing there.

Mom Tip of the Week:
When discouragement creeps in, look for tiny signs of growth: a smile, a moment of calm, a new skill, a small answered prayer. These little glimpses are reminders that a beautiful harvest is on the way.

Give Thanks Always

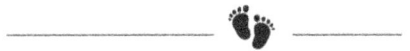

"Give thanks in all circumstances; for this is God's will for you in Christ Jesus."
-1 Thessalonians 5:18

Gratitude has a beautiful way of softening even the hardest days of motherhood. It doesn't demand that you deny your exhaustion or pretend things are perfect. Instead, it invites you to pause long enough to notice the small fingerprints of God's grace woven into your everyday life.

Some days feel heavy, naps don't happen, plans unravel, and the house looks like a storm rolled through. But even in those messy moments, God is moving. When you choose to say, "Thank You, Lord," something shifts inside you. Your perspective steadies. Your heart lifts. Weariness begins to turn into worship.

Gratitude doesn't ignore the hard parts; it simply reminds you that God is present in all of it. It helps you see the sacred in the simple, the sweetness of your baby's smile, the comfort of a warm cup of tea, the strength that helps you stand back up when you feel worn thin.

These "little" gifts aren't little at all; they're daily reminders of His love.

And here's the beautiful thing: giving thanks in all circumstances isn't about the circumstances, it's about trusting the God who walks through them with you. Gratitude won't always change the situation, but it will always change *you*. It fills your spirit with peace, joy, and a deep awareness that you are never alone.

Prayer:

Lord, thank You for the goodness You pour into my life, even on the days when I struggle to see it. Open my eyes to the small blessings that remind me You're near. Teach me to carry a thankful heart in every circumstance, and let my gratitude draw me closer to You. Amen.

Challenge of the Week:
Each night, speak three things out loud that you're grateful for, whether it's a quiet moment, a lesson learned, or simply making it through the day. Gratitude grows when it's voiced.

Mom Tip of the Week:
Start a "thankful jar." Write down moments of blessing, even tiny ones, and tuck them inside. On difficult days, pull out a few and remind your heart of God's steady, faithful goodness.

Julie Whitecotton

Joy in Every Season

"I have learned to be content whatever the circumstances."
- Philippians 4:11

Motherhood comes in waves of seasons, some sweet, some stretching, and some that leave you wondering if you're doing any of it right. One day you're savoring baby giggles and tiny milestones, and the next you're counting the minutes until bedtime, praying for strength you don't feel you have. It's so easy in these moments to long for the next stage: a full night's sleep, a calmer routine, a little more "you" time. But joy doesn't wait for the next season. Joy meets you right where you are.

Paul wrote about contentment while walking through one of the hardest chapters of his life. His joy didn't come from comfort, it came from trust. And that same truth holds power for you. When you stop believing that things need to be perfect to be meaningful, your heart becomes free to notice joy in the simple, ordinary moments.

Joy shows up in the early morning snuggles, in the quiet places where you whisper prayers no one else hears, in the small victories that remind you God is gently guiding you. This season, with all its challenges, all its surprises, all its beauty, is part of God's story for you. He isn't just carrying you through it; He's shaping you in it.

Every stage of motherhood has its own kind of wonder. When you look for joy, even intentionally for a few seconds each day, you'll begin to see that God's goodness is woven into your ordinary moments. Joy doesn't depend on how easy the day is; it depends on the God who never changes.

Prayer:

Lord, thank You for the steady joy You offer in every season of my life. Slow my heart when I'm tempted to rush ahead or wish away the day. Help me see the beauty You've placed right in front of me and to be content in the season You've chosen for me. Fill my heart with Your joy today. Amen.

Challenge of the Week:

Each evening, recall one joyful moment from the day, even something small, and thank God for it before you fall asleep.

Mom Tip of the Week:

Take a weekly "real-life" photo, not the perfect shot, but the true one. These little snapshots will one day remind you how much joy lived inside this beautifully ordinary season.

Be a Light

"You are the light of the world. A town built on a hill cannot be hidden."
- Matthew 5:14

Motherhood often takes place in the quiet corners of life in midnight feedings, whispered prayers, messy kitchens, and moments that rarely get noticed or celebrated. And yet, Jesus speaks directly into those hidden spaces and reminds you: *You are the light of the world.* Not someday... not when things feel easier... not when you finally feel "put together." You're a light *right now*.

Your light shines in ways you may not even realize. It shines when you choose patience over irritation, when you speak gently even though you're tired, when you comfort your child with tenderness, and when you love your family with a faithful, steady heart. These aren't small things. They are holy things, glimpses of Jesus shining through you.

And here's the beautiful truth: your light doesn't have to be big or perfect to matter. God uses simple, everyday acts of love to brighten the lives around you. The world is desperate for gentleness, compassion, and hope, and God has placed you right where you are to reflect those things. Your life becomes a quiet testimony: a reminder that God is faithful, present, and loving, even in the busiest or most exhausting seasons.

But there will be days when you feel dim when exhaustion, discouragement, or overwhelm make your light feel faint. On those days, don't try to shine harder. Come back to the Source. Sit with God, even for a moment. Let His love refill you, restore you, and reignite the flame inside your heart. As His light fills you, it naturally flows out into your home and into the people you touch.

You are a light not because you're trying to be, but because God placed His light inside you.

Prayer:

Lord, thank You for calling me to be a light in my home and in the world. When I feel tired or unnoticed, remind me that even the smallest acts of love shine brightly in Your eyes. Fill me with Your Spirit today. Rekindle my strength, renew my joy, and let Your light shine through every word and action. Amen.

Challenge of the Week:

Choose one intentional act of kindness this week: a note, a prayer, a small gift, or a helping hand, and ask God to use it to reflect His love to someone who needs it.

Mom Tip of the Week:

Light spreads through simple gestures. A smile, a kind word, or a quiet prayer for someone can brighten not just their day, but yours too. Small kindnesses create a big impact.

Julie Whitecotton

Faithful and True

"The One who calls you is faithful,
and He will do it."
-1 Thessalonians 5:24

Motherhood comes with so many promises you make to your baby, to yourself, and even silently to God. You promise to be patient, to stay calm, to always do your best. But as the days unfold, you quickly discover that you're human. There are moments when you forget something important, moments when your patience wears thin, and moments when you feel like you're falling short of the mother you hoped to be. And yet... God remains faithful.

Where your strength ends, His begins. Where you feel inconsistent, He is steady. The God who invited you into motherhood didn't accidentally place this calling on your life. He chose you with full knowledge of your strengths *and* your struggles. He knew you would have exhausted nights, overwhelmed mornings, and days when you'd question whether you're doing enough. And even so, He called you because He promised to be your strength, your guide, and your help.

His faithfulness shows up in countless ways:
- in the peace that suddenly calms your heart,
- in the strength that carries you through another long night,
- in the joy that appears unexpectedly in the middle of an ordinary day.

He is faithful in the big miracles and faithful in the tiny, unnoticed ones, the ones hidden in diaper changes, whispered prayers, and rocking-chair moments when you wonder if anyone sees. He sees. And He is with you.

Motherhood isn't about being perfect; it's about trusting the One who *is* perfect. He will finish the work He started in you. When you feel inadequate, remind yourself that God is more than enough.

Prayer:

Lord, thank You for being faithful even when I feel unsure or overwhelmed. When I fall short, remind me that You never fail. Help me trust that You are working in me and through me, one moment at a time. Strengthen my heart today with the assurance that You called me to this role and You will carry me through it. Amen.

Challenge of the Week:

Each day, pause and thank God for one moment where His faithfulness was clear: a provision, a peaceful moment, a kind word, a burst of strength, or an answered prayer.

Mom Tip of the Week:

When doubts whisper in your mind, speak this truth aloud: *"God is faithful. He called me. He will help me."* Let His faithfulness quiet every fear.

God's Love Endures

"Give thanks to the Lord, for He is good;
His love endures forever."
-Psalm 100:5

Motherhood will give you days that fill your heart to the brim... and days that empty you. There are moments when your patience feels stretched thin, when your heart feels tired, or when you wonder if anyone truly sees how much you're carrying. But in every emotion, in the joy and in the heaviness, one truth remains unshakably steady: God's love for you never changes.

His love doesn't rise and fall with your mood or your performance. It doesn't weaken when you feel overwhelmed or frustrated. It doesn't disappear on the days you feel like you're barely holding on. His love endures steady, faithful, and unbroken through every season of your motherhood and every moment of your life.

On the days when you feel unseen, God sees you. On the days when you feel unappreciated, He values you. On the days when you feel worn down, He holds you closer.

Just as you love your child through tears, tantrums, messes, and midnight wake-ups, God loves you fully, deeply, and unwaveringly. You don't lose His love when you lose your patience. You don't lessen His love when you make mistakes. His love is not fragile. It doesn't depend on your effort. It's anchored in who He is, good, constant, everlasting.

And as you pour love into your child day after day, remember that you are living out a reflection of His heart. You're giving a human picture of the kind of love God lavishes on you: enduring, compassionate, faithful. Let that truth be the shelter your heart returns to, especially when the day feels long and your confidence feels thin.

You are held. You are loved. You are never forgotten.

Prayer:

Lord, thank You for a love that doesn't fade with my feelings or failures. When I feel tired, discouraged, or uncertain, remind me that I am wrapped in Your never-ending love. Help me rest in that truth and let it overflow into how I love my child and those around me. Amen.

Challenge of the Week:
Write this truth somewhere you will see it often: "God's love endures forever even for me." Read it aloud whenever your heart needs comfort.

Mom Tip of the Week:
End each day by thanking God for one way He showed His love through peace, strength, a small blessing, or a simple moment of joy. Gratitude prepares your heart to rest in His unchanging love.

Julie Whitecotton

Hope Shines Bright

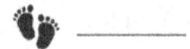

"May the God of hope fill you with all joy and peace as you trust in Him, so that you may overflow with hope by the power of the Holy Spirit."
-Romans 15:13

Some seasons of motherhood feel long and heavy. The days blur together, the nights stretch on, and sometimes you wonder if you'll ever feel fully rested again. It's in those moments when your body is tired and your heart feels stretched thin that hope can seem far away.

But God's hope is different from the kind the world offers. It isn't fragile. Your circumstances don't limit it. It doesn't flicker out when life feels overwhelming.

God's hope is steady because it's rooted in who He is: faithful, present, and unchanging.

You don't have to manufacture your own hope or pretend you're okay. God never asked you to be strong on your own. Instead, He pours hope into you through the Holy Spirit, the kind of hope that lifts your chin, softens your heart, and reminds you that you are not walking this season alone.

Even a tiny spark of hope can change the way you see your day. It doesn't erase the hard parts, but it shines light into them. It helps you notice the holy moments tucked inside the ordinary ones, the sleepy smiles, the quiet snuggles, the unexpected peace in the middle of chaos.

God didn't bring you this far to leave you here. He is still working, still guiding, still carrying you.

Let this truth anchor you: light always returns. Even the longest night has a sunrise.

Julie Whitecotton

Prayer:

Lord, thank You for being the God of hope that doesn't fade when I'm tired or discouraged. When my days feel heavy, fill me again with Your joy and Your peace. Let Your light shine in me and through me, reminding me that I am never alone. Amen.

Challenge of the Week:

Each morning, speak one simple truth out loud before the day begins, something like, *"God is with me,"* or *"Hope is rising,"* or *"Better days are ahead."* Let those words shape your heart before anything else does.

Mom Tip of the Week:

Place a small candle or a string of soft lights somewhere you can see them during the day. Let it be a gentle reminder: even when life feels dim, God's hope is still shining.

Guided by His Light

"Your word is a lamp to my feet and a light to my path."
-Psalm 119:105

Motherhood doesn't come with a rulebook or step-by-step instructions. Some days you feel confident and steady, and other days you're standing in the middle of decisions that feel too big, too heavy, or too unfamiliar. Moments arise when you wonder, *"Am I doing this right? Am I choosing the best for my child?"*

It can feel a little like walking through fog, you can't see very far ahead, and every step takes courage.

But God hasn't left you to wander blindly. He has given you His Word not as a spotlight that reveals the whole future, but as a soft, steady lamp that guides you one step at a time. And sometimes, that's all you need.

When the day feels confusing, when emotions swirl, or when the noise of life makes it hard to think clearly, returning to Scripture quiets the heart. God's Word nourishes your spirit. It settles your thoughts. It brings a peace that isn't rooted in knowing every answer, but in knowing the One who does.

As you spend time with Him, even in small moments, even with interruptions, you'll begin to notice His gentle guidance in your everyday life. A whisper to slow down. A reminder to breathe. A nudge to trust instead of panic. His light doesn't push you; it leads you kindly. You don't have to be a perfect mom to walk in His light. You have to stay close to the Source.

Step by step, decision by decision, He will faithfully guide you through the joy, the uncertainty, and every season still ahead.

Prayer:

Lord, thank You for Your Word that steadies my heart when I feel unsure. When my path feels unclear, draw me back to Your presence. Light the steps in front of me, and help me trust Your guidance more than my fears. Walk with me as I walk with my child. Amen.

Challenge of the Week:

Each morning this week, pause to read one verse, even just a single line of Scripture, and ask God, *"How can I live this today?"* Let His Word shape your heart before anything else speaks into your day.

Mom Tip of the Week:

Choose a verse that brings peace and write it somewhere you'll see often, taped to the mirror, on your fridge, or as your phone's lock screen. Let God's light meet you right where you are.

Julie Whitecotton

Moments of Renewal

"But those who hope in the Lord will renew their strength. They will soar on wings like eagles; they will run and not grow weary, they will walk and not be faint."
-Isaiah 40:31

Motherhood is wonderful, but let's be honest, it can also drain you in ways you didn't know were possible. You give and give, often without a break, until you suddenly realize your tank is running low. Some days you wake up tired, and by the afternoon, you're wondering how you'll have enough strength for the rest of the day.

But God sees your exhaustion, and He does not leave you there. He promises renewal, not just a little boost of energy, but real, deep restoration that touches your body, your mind, and your spirit.

And here's the gentle truth: renewal doesn't always show up in dramatic "mountaintop" moments. More often, God slips it quietly into your day in a calm breath while your baby sleeps on your chest, in a whispered prayer while folding laundry, in a moment of clarity when you remember that you're not alone.

When you pause long enough to look toward Him instead of pushing yourself harder, something beautiful happens: His strength takes the place of your striving. His peace begins to cover the places where worry used to sit. You don't have to feel strong to receive His strength; you have to be willing to lean on Him.

And remember this: God is not expecting you to soar every single day. Some days, soaring will happen. Other days, simply walking slowly, faithfully, will be enough. He honors both. He carries you when you cannot carry yourself, and He holds you steady until your wings are ready to rise again.

Prayer:

Lord, thank You for Your promise to renew my strength. When I feel empty or weary, remind me to turn toward You instead of trying to push through on my own. Fill the tired places in my heart with Your peace. Restore me so I can love from a place of overflow, not exhaustion. Amen.

Challenge of the Week:

Choose one moment each day, even just a couple of minutes, to pause. Sit, breathe deeply, whisper a prayer, or step outside for fresh air. Let that moment be your invitation for God to renew you before you continue your day.

Mom Tip of the Week:

Don't wait for a long break to recharge. Sometimes, the quietest, smallest pause with God restores more than an entire day of trying to "escape" ever could.

Steadfast in Spirit

"Create in me a clean heart, O God, and renew a steadfast spirit within me."
-Psalm 51:10

Motherhood is always shifting. When you adjust to one stage, another one arrives. One day, you feel like you've got a good rhythm, and the next day everything feels upside down, your emotions, your patience, even your confidence.

It's completely normal to feel unsteady at times. But God never intended for your stability to come from routines or predictability. He invites you to anchor your heart in Him, the One who never changes.

A steadfast spirit doesn't mean you walk around unbothered or unaffected. It means that even when the day feels chaotic, your heart is rooted in something deeper than the chaos. When guilt tries to whisper lies, when comparison steals your joy, when frustration rises quicker than you'd like, that is exactly when God says, *Come to Me. Let Me renew you from the inside out.*

Every time you invite God into your day, He clears away the things that tangle your heart: worry, frustration, and self-doubt, and

He replaces them with peace, patience, and clarity. Steadfastness grows in those small, quiet conversations with Him, the whispered prayers over the sink, the Scripture you hold onto while you rock your baby, the deep breath that becomes a surrender.

Over time, you'll notice something beautiful: the same situations that once shook you no longer carry the same power. Not because life got easier, but because your spirit grew stronger. A mother rooted in God's presence is not easily moved.

Prayer:

Lord, renew my heart today and steady my spirit. When I feel overwhelmed or unsure, remind me that You are constant even when my day is not. Anchor my thoughts in Your truth and fill me with Your peace. Make my spirit strong, calm, and grounded in You. Amen.

Challenge of the Week:

Begin each morning with this simple prayer: "Lord, make my heart steady and my spirit strong." Whisper it again any time your peace feels shaky.

Mom Tip of the Week:

Choose one verse that brings your heart comfort and place it somewhere you'll see often, above the sink, on your phone screen, or by your baby's changing table. Let God's Word recalibrate your spirit throughout the day.

Julie Whitecotton

Overflowing with Gratitude

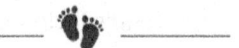

*"Give thanks to the Lord, for He is good;
His love endures forever."*

-Psalm 107:1

Gratitude has this gentle, quiet power to reshape your whole day. It doesn't magically erase the hard moments of motherhood, but it softens them. It shifts your eyes from what's overwhelming to what's overflowing. And the truth is, even on the messiest, most exhausting days, God's goodness is still woven through your life. Sometimes gratitude looks simply:

The way your baby leans into you, the tiny fingers wrapped around yours, the hush that fills the house after bedtime, the strength you didn't know you had until you needed it.

These little moments are God's fingerprints, reminders that His love is in the details, not just the big breakthroughs.

But as a mom, it's also easy to get caught in the swirl of everything that feels unfinished: the dishes, the responsibilities, the prayers you're still waiting to see answered. Gratitude gently slows that swirl. It asks you to pause. To breathe. To look around at all God has already done.

And here's the beautiful part: When your heart leans toward gratitude, it naturally leaves less room for worry, comparison, or frustration. You start to see life not through the lens of lack, but through the fullness of God's love.

Gratitude isn't just something you feel, it's something you practice. It's whispering "thank you" before you even roll out of bed. It's noticing a blessing in the middle of a hard moment. It's remembering that every good thing comes from a God whose love never shifts, never weakens, and never ends.

As you practice this rhythm of thankfulness, your child will grow up learning it too, not because of what you say, but because of what you live. And that, mama, is a legacy worth passing on.

Prayer:

Lord, thank You for Your goodness that meets me in every season. Teach me to live with a heart that notices Your blessings, even on my hardest days. Help gratitude rise in me until it spills into everything I do. Let thankfulness be my daily song and my steady anchor. Amen.

Challenge of the Week:

Start a gratitude chain this week. Each day, write one thing you're thankful for on a small strip of paper and link them together. Watch it grow as a visual reminder of how faithful God has been.

Mom Tip of the Week:

When you feel the weight of the day pressing on you, stop for just a moment and thank God for *one thing right where you are*. That simple shift can quiet stress and make space for peace.

Grace-Filled Growth

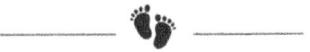

*"But grow in the grace and knowledge of
our Lord and Savior Jesus Christ."*
-2 Peter 3:18

Motherhood is one of the greatest classrooms God will ever place you in. Every day brings something new, new joys, new challenges, new opportunities to stretch in ways you didn't know were possible. Some days you feel like you're handling it all beautifully; other days, you feel like you're learning everything from scratch. But here's the good news: God is growing you through it all... even on the days when you don't feel it.

His grace is not just what saves you, it's what shapes you. Grace is what meets you when you lose your patience, what steadies you when you feel overwhelmed, and what gently whispers, *"You're still growing, and that's okay."*

It's so easy as a mom to look back over the day and focus on what you could've done better, the tone you wish you hadn't used, the moment you felt frustrated, the tasks you couldn't finish. But God isn't tallying your mistakes. He's tending to your growth. He knows every challenge you face and uses each one as a tool to deepen your character and strengthen your spirit.

Just like your baby grows little by little, often in ways you only notice later, you're growing too. Every time you choose compassion over irritation, every breath you take instead of reacting, every prayer you whisper in the middle of a long day... that's growth. Real, holy, grace-filled growth.

You don't have to rush it. You don't have to get it perfect. Growth in God's kingdom is slow, steady, and anchored in His love. Be gentle with yourself. God is patient with you, and He invites you to extend that same grace to yourself.

Prayer:

Lord, thank You for Your grace that meets me exactly where I am. When I feel discouraged or inadequate, remind me that You are still shaping me, day by day. Help me to grow with patience, humility, and trust. Teach me to offer myself the same grace You so freely pour out. Amen.

Challenge of the Week:

Think about one area where you've grown since becoming a mom, patience, confidence, faith, or even your ability to laugh instead of stress. Write it down and thank God for the quiet ways He's been shaping your heart.

Mom Tip of the Week:

Don't look for perfection, look for progress. Every small step you take in love, patience, and faithfulness matters more than you realize.

Julie Whitecotton

The Power of Perseverance

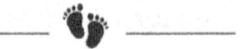

"Let perseverance finish its work so that you may be mature and complete, not lacking anything."
-James 1:4

Motherhood is truly a long-distance journey. It's not about sprinting through perfect days, it's about showing up again and again, even when your energy is low and your patience feels thin. There are days when it seems like everything is happening at once, the crying, the dishes, the errands, the emotions, and you wonder how much more you can give. But it's in these very moments that God is building something strong and lasting within you.

Perseverance in motherhood isn't about pushing yourself beyond your limits or pretending you're fine. It's about continuing forward while leaning on the One who never grows tired. God isn't asking you to be superhuman; He's inviting you to rely on His strength. Every time you choose love when you're exhausted, every time you whisper a prayer in frustration, every time you take a deep breath and keep going, you are living out perseverance.

And here's the beautiful part: God never wastes these moments. He uses them to shape your heart in ways you may not see yet. You're becoming more patient, more compassionate, more resilient, not because life is easy, but because His grace is at work in you. The qualities He's cultivating through your perseverance will bless your child, your home, and even your future self.

So, on the days when the load feels heavy, remember this truth: you're not just enduring... you're growing. You're becoming. And God is right beside you, giving you strength for each step.

Prayer:

Lord, thank You for the strength You provide each day. When I feel tired or overwhelmed, remind me that You are shaping me through these moments. Help me lean on You and keep moving forward with grace and faith. Finish the work You've begun in me. Amen.

Challenge of the Week:

When a difficult moment comes, pause and softly pray, *"God, give me the strength to keep going."* Let that simple prayer anchor your heart and redirect your focus.

Mom Tip of the Week:

You don't have to be perfect, just present. Showing up consistently, even imperfectly, is what builds strong homes and strong hearts.

Strength in Unity

"Though one may be overpowered, two can defend themselves. A cord of three strands is not quickly broken."
-Ecclesiastes 4:12

Motherhood can be beautiful, but it can also feel unbelievably lonely at times. You can be surrounded by noise, tiny hands, and a full house and still feel like you're carrying the entire weight of life on your own. The quiet moments after a long day, the unspoken worries, the mental load you juggle... it can leave you feeling isolated even in a room full of people.

But God never meant for you to walk this path alone. From the very beginning, He designed you for connection for support, for friendship, for community. And not just human connection, but connection with Him at the very center of it all. When your relationships are woven together with His strength, they become like a thick, braided cord strong enough to withstand anything that comes your way.

God often uses people to hold us up:
- A spouse who whispers, "You're doing great."
- A friend who listens without judgment.
- A fellow mom who says, "I've been there too."
- A parent or sibling who steps in at just the right time.

Asking for help isn't a sign of weakness, it's humility, courage, and wisdom. It's allowing others to be the hands and feet of Jesus in your life. When you open your heart and let people in, you experience the kind of unity God designed: grace-giving, burden-sharing, prayer-filled community.

But the strongest unity you will ever experience is when God Himself is woven into your relationships. When he is the third strand in your marriage, your friendships, your motherhood, suddenly your support system becomes unbreakable. He strengthens the bonds, deepens the love, and gives stability even when life feels anything but stable.

You were never meant to do this alone, mama. Let others walk with you. Let God stand at the center. Together, you will find the strength you never knew you had.

Prayer:

Lord, thank You for the people You've placed in my life. Help me open my heart to their support and be a source of encouragement in return. Strengthen every relationship with Your love and bind us together in unity that cannot be shaken. Walk with me through every season, and remind me that I am never alone. Amen.

Challenge of the Week:

Reach out to someone who has encouraged your faith, a friend, a mentor, or a fellow mom. Send them a message, a prayer, or a simple "thank you" for walking beside you.

Mom Tip of the Week:

Motherhood becomes lighter when shared. Don't hesitate to ask for help; allowing others to support you is one of the ways God shows His love and care.

Julie Whitecotton

A Heart of Joy

"The joy of the Lord is your strength."
-Nehemiah 8:10

Motherhood is an emotional journey, sometimes overflowing with laughter and sweetness, and other times marked by exhaustion, overwhelm, or even tears you didn't expect to shed. There are days when joy feels effortless, like it rises naturally from your heart. And then there are days when joy feels distant, like something you have to chase but can't quite grasp.

But here's the beautiful truth: your joy doesn't start with your circumstances; it starts with God. His joy is steady, constant, and unshaken by sleepless nights, messy rooms, or tough moments. It's a joy that anchors you when everything around you feels uncertain. It's a strength that doesn't depend on how well the day is going, but on who He is.

Joy often shows up in the small, sacred moments
- the sound of your baby's giggle,
- the warmth of a sleepy snuggle,
- the quiet of early morning,
- the deep breath you didn't know you needed.

Those little glimpses are reminders that God is near. But even when joy feels harder to find, He's still right there offering His own joy to fill the places where yours feels thin. His joy is a fruit of His Spirit, gently growing in you day by day, even in seasons when you feel anything but strong.

And here's the beautiful connection: joy gives strength. Not the loud, energetic kind but the steady, quiet strength that helps you keep showing up, keep loving, keep pushing through the messy and the mundane with grace. Joy doesn't deny the hard parts of motherhood; it simply invites God into them. It reminds you that His presence is greater than any challenge you're facing.

Let His joy settle into your heart today, not as a feeling you must force, but as a gift you can receive.

Prayer:

Lord, thank You for being the steady source of my joy. On the days when my spirit feels heavy or tired, draw me close and fill me with Your strength. Help me see moments of joy in the middle of my busy, messy days. Let my heart rest in the happiness that comes from knowing You are with me. Amen.

Challenge of the Week:

Each day, notice one small thing that brings you joy, a moment, a sound, a smile, a breath, and thank God for it. Write them down throughout the week to remind yourself that joy is always present when your heart looks for it.

Mom Tip of the Week:

Begin your mornings with a simple smile, even before the coffee and the chaos of the day. A joyful, grateful heart doesn't just strengthen you... It shapes the atmosphere of your home and blesses your little one, too.

A Year of Grace

"The Lord has done great things for us, and we are filled with joy."
-Psalm 126:3

You've made it through an entire year of motherhood, a year filled with moments that changed you forever. A year of first cries, first smiles, first steps of faith as you learned how to care for this precious little life. A year of letting go, growing up, leaning in, and sometimes breaking down... only to find God right there, lifting you back up again.

Looking back, you may realize that the greatest transformation didn't just happen in your baby, it happened in you. You've discovered strength you didn't know you had. You've learned a love deeper than anything you imagined. You've embraced grace in ways you never needed before.

And all of it, every high and every low, has been held together by the steady faithfulness of God.

There were days you whispered, *"I can't do this anymore."* And yet... You did. There were nights you sat in the dark, exhausted and overwhelmed. And somehow, morning always came. That isn't luck or coincidence, that's the gentle, unfailing hand of your Father carrying you.

He saw every tear, heard every prayer, and filled every gap where your strength ran out. He walked with you through fear, through joy, through confusion, through laughter. And He didn't just help you survive this year, He helped you grow through it.

As you step into a new season, remember this: Motherhood was never meant to be about perfection. It's about presence. Your presence with your child... And God's presence with you.

You don't have to master every stage before you get there. You take it day by day with the One who has already prepared the road ahead. The God who began this beautiful work in your heart, in your home, and in your child's life *will* be faithful to continue it.

So, breathe deeply, mama. You've come so far, and with God, the best is still ahead.

Prayer:

Lord, thank You for walking with me through this first year of motherhood. Thank You for Your strength when I felt weak, Your peace when anxiety crept in, and Your joy woven through every season. As I step into the days ahead, help me carry Your grace with me, steadying me, guiding me, and filling my heart with hope. Amen.

Challenge of the Week:

Set aside a few quiet minutes to reflect on how God has shown up for you this year. Write a letter of gratitude to Him, to your baby, or even to yourself, celebrating the growth, the grace, and the goodness you've experienced.

Mom Tip of the Week:

Celebrate this milestone. Celebrate the victories, the breakthroughs, the messy moments you survived, and the beauty you created along the way. You've grown. Your baby has flourished. And God has been faithful through it all. Take time to rest, rejoice, and thank Him for this incredible journey.

Closing

As you come to the end of this 52-week journey, pause for a moment and breathe. Look back at where you started and notice just how much God has brought you through. You've survived sleepless nights, whispered prayers in the dark, and days when you weren't sure you had anything left to give. And yet... You made it. Not because everything was easy, but because God was faithful every single step of the way.

Think of all the tiny moments you didn't realize were shaping you: the late-night feedings, the tears wiped away, the quiet moments when you held your baby close and asked God for strength. Those weren't just tasks or struggles. They were holy places where God met you, shaped you, and grew something beautiful inside you.

Motherhood will keep shifting as your child grows, and the seasons ahead will bring new joys and new challenges. But one thing will remain constant: God's grace will always be enough for you. The same grace that carried you through this year will carry you through every year to come.

When you feel uncertain, return to the Word that steadied your heart before. When you're unsure of what to do next, remember the God who guided you through sleepless nights, anxious thoughts, and unexpected blessings. He hasn't changed, and He never will.

Your journey is bigger than diapers, schedules, and routines. You're not just raising a child, you're sowing seeds of faith. Every cuddle, every prayer, every act of patience, every moment of grace, it's all part of the legacy you are building. A legacy God is incredibly proud of.

So, as you step forward from here, may you carry this truth with you:
- You are loved.
- You are chosen.
- You are never walking alone.
-

No matter what season you enter next, may your heart stay anchored in His peace, your spirit grounded in His hope, and your days filled with reminders of His unfailing love.

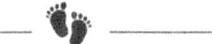

"The Lord will guide you always;
He will satisfy your needs in a sun-scorched land.
And will strengthen your frame.
You will be like a well-watered garden, like a spring whose waters never fail."

- Isaiah 58:11

Julie Whitecotton

Scripture quotations taken from the *Holy Bible, New International Version®, NIV®.*
Copyright ©1973, 1978, 1984, 2011 by Biblica, Inc.™
Used by permission of Zondervan. All rights reserved worldwide.
www.zondervan.com
The "NIV" and "New International Version" are trademarks registered in the United States Patent and Trademark Office by Biblica, Inc.™

Scripture taken from the New King James Version®. Copyright © 1982 by Thomas Nelson. Used by permission. All rights reserved.

Printed in the United States of America

Made in the USA
Coppell, TX
29 January 2026

70243726R20095